Fixing Bunions Without Surgery

How To Avoid Having Feet Like Your Mother

by Daniel Fitzpatrick

B.App.SC (Pod) M.A.Pod A

International #1 Best Seller

Amazon #1 Best Selling Book in 4 Countries and 5 Categories

evolve Global Publishing
www.evolveglobalpublishing.com.au

COPYRIGHT

Daniel Fitzpatrick, Shop 6, 27 Belgrave Street, Manly, NSW, 2095

Website: www.alternativefootsolutions.com.au
Email: info@alternativefootsolutions.com.au
Phone: 02 8966 9300 or +61 2 8966 9300

Ordering Information: Quantity sales. Special discounts are available on multiple purchases by corporations, associations, and others.

For details, contact the "Special Sales Department" at the address above.

Alternative Foot Solutions, Daniel Fitzpatrick --1st edition, 2016

First Published 2016 for Daniel Fitzpatrick by Evolve Global Publishing
PO Box 327 Stanhope Gardens NSW 2768
info@evolveglobalpublishing.com
www.evolveglobalpublishing.com

evolve Global Publishing
www.evolveglobalpublishing.com.au

Book Layout: © 2016 Evolve Global Publishing

ISBN: (Paperback) 978-1-945173-85-1

ISBN: (Hardback) 978-1-945176-43-2

ISBN-13: (Createspace) 978-1533246-58-5

ISBN-10: (Createspace) 1533246580

ISBN: (Smashwords) 978-1-311386-10-6

ASIN: (Amazon Kindle) B01C04AHFQ

This book is available on Barnes & Noble, Kobo, Apple iBooks (digital), Google Books (digital)

Table of Contents

Foreword

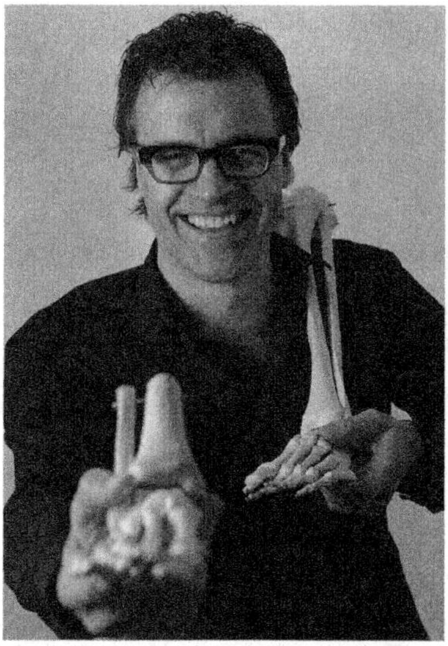

Finally, the book that I always wanted to write has now been written!

Thank you, Daniel, for getting this crucial message into the public domain where it needs to be heard. So many bunion sufferers will benefit from this book.

I've known Daniel since 2002 when he first trained with me in Foot Mobilisation Therapies (FMT) in Adelaide, South Australia. I vividly recall Daniel's enthusiasm, his inquisitive mind and dedication to helping his patients get better clinical outcomes for their health.

Daniel's commitment to providing the highest quality professional services to his patients has not diminished in the time I've known him. It's made him a stellar practitioner of the highest caliber. His patients are fortunate to receive some of the best quality of care in Australia.

Daniel has focused his considerable expertise to helping his patients with bunions get back to enjoying their life. Not only that, he's helped thousands of patients avoid surgery. This is a remarkable achievement and one that he should be proud of.

This book is just a small cross section of the wide variety of people Daniel has helped. I know that many more people will also benefit as a result of receiving the wisdom that is packed into this book. Daniel has boiled down complex biomechanical and physiological concepts into understandable content that is easy to read and grasp.

Daniel has courageously voiced his opinions and experiences based on thousands of clinical cases. His book will challenge the conservative medical establishment and ruffle feathers. To Daniel's credit he has never been shy of controversy and has been willing to stick his neck out so that many more people with bunions will benefit.

If you or someone you care about suffers with bunions, then make sure they read this book because it could save them from years of unnecessary suffering. Daniel's book is chock full of practical tips and real world case studies that any bunion sufferer can benefit from.

This book is a 'world first' because it's patient-centric and works to help bunion sufferers reduce their suffering. Daniel's clinical experience shines through the pages of this book as he generously gives of his wisdom to help others.

Enjoy this book and pass it on to someone else who can also benefit. Please spread the word that there are safe and effective alternatives to bunion surgery.

Ted Jedynak
Podiatrist & International Educator

Ted has specialised in Foot Mobilisation Techniques (FMT) exclusively since 1996.

ABOUT THE AUTHOR

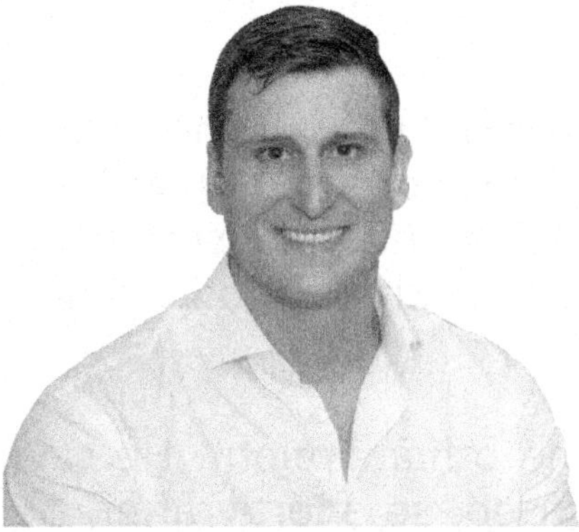

Daniel Fitzpatrick is a #1 international best-selling Australian author, public speaker, and he's a successful, qualified podiatrist. He has written a number of articles, and moreover, he has made guest appearances on TV, including Channel 9's A Current Affair, Channel 7's Today Tonight.

He also featured in Good Health Magazine. In addition, Daniel is a popular speaker at industry conferences. As a clinician, Daniel's main work involves directing, consulting and overseeing Alternative Foot Solutions, which is a very successful podiatry practice in Sydney, Australia, which specialises in Foot Mobilisation Therapy; this service is unique in New South Wales, as no other clinic specialises in these treatments.

Daniel lives at Sydney Northern Beaches with his wife and son; he loves to surf and is a very active person.

One of the main reasons Daniel chose podiatry was because he was treated by an excellent podiatrist when he was younger, and it made such a positive impression that he decided to pursue a career in the field. Daniel qualified as a podiatrist (BappSc (Pod) M.A.Pod A.) in 2002 at the University of Western Sydney.

The first year after he graduated university and started practicing podiatry, Daniel had a number of consecutive female patients who presented to him in a short space of time, all in a distressed state.

There was one female patient in particular who presented in a very frustrated state after he had fitted her into a pair of orthotics a month earlier. She was quite distraught, because despite spending many hundreds of dollars on a set of orthotics, she could no longer fit into her shoes.

The discussion escalated into a disagreement about shoes, and she became quite emotional about it. She expressed frustration about not being able to wear shoes that simultaneously looked good and assuaged her foot pain, because the orthotics didn't fit into her shoes.

Daniel thought: "There must be some other option". He saw a course on foot mobilisation advertised, so shortly after, he completed one of those courses. On the first day of the course, he thought: "This is quite amazing".

After doing that first set of training, he was extremely impressed with the results, so he started to treat a whole range of people using the methods he had learned in the training. He treated each patient far more extensively than what he needed to, and for the first six months, he actually treated a whole group of people free of charge to ensure it worked.

What he soon found was not only was the treatment better, it was far superior to orthotics, and most impressively, compliance levels were through the roof.

His patients were extremely happy, and his working existence was rendered much more enjoyable. By that stage, bunions had become an extremely prevalent issue.

No-one had an option for treating bunions, so his thinking was that if foot mobilisation could realign the rest of your foot, why couldn't it realign your big toe?

Daniel and his team started developing their techniques so they could treat bunions more effectively. With great success, he started treating every bunion that he saw with Foot Mobilisation Therapy. The result was that he had much happier patients and much better outcomes with his treatments, not to mention, a much higher compliance level.

He was so busy with Foot Mobilisation that it quickly became clear it was a better use of his time and resources to open his own clinic where he just focused on Foot Mobilisation Therapy.

Daniel's core business is foot mobilisation therapy, and he and his team are the only people in New South Wales who currently do it. In fact, there are only four other people within the country who provide this service to the same level that they provide it.

The major benefit of their service is that they are able to treat and fix feet to help their clients avoid surgery and orthotics. One of the key advantages of the type of treatment they provide is that it opens up much broader footwear options for females.

After visiting their surgery for their initial consultation, it is not unusual for people to cancel their scheduled bunion surgery soon after. They've saved themselves thousands of dollars. It's self-evident then why Daniel and his team are keen to get the word out to people who're currently living with painful, untreated bunions.

Nevertheless, Daniel contends that most surgeons are very ethical in terms of discouraging unnecessary and potentially damaging surgery, so they must be given credit. Daniel commented: "Most of the good ones with whom we interact tend not to be proponents of Foot Mobilisation, but by the same token, they will invariably try to talk people out of surgery as much as possible, because most good surgeons have no shortage of patients".

The success of this treatment is explained by the fact that Daniel addresses the underlying cause; he changes the actual alignment of the patients' joints, and then he also strengthens the muscles around it.

This, in turn, stimulates the nervous system to change the neural patterns and gate patterns to reinforce that positive position. Anything else is a band-aid approach when it comes to treating bunions, and this includes orthotics.

Unlike Foot Mobilisation Therapy, orthotics fail to address the underlying cause of the bunion.

INTRODUCTION

Are you a fashionable woman with a bunion?

Wear the shoes you love, without undergoing surgery!
Almost 40% of the population of Australia will suffer some sort of problem with their feet during their lifetime. Something as simple as a toenail infection can be treated with antiseptic creams and professional trimming, whereas more complex problems, such as bunions, are likely to require orthotics, or in more severe cases, surgery to relieve the symptoms.

Problems in the feet can cause pain and stress in seemingly unrelated areas of the body. To understand why so many of us suffer from foot problems, let me first explain a bit about the complex structure of the human foot.The foot and ankle contain 26 bones. One-quarter of the bones in the human body are in the feet.

The foot has a total of 33 joints, and more than 100 muscles, tendons and ligaments, including a network of blood vessels, nerves, skin, and soft tissue.

The average person will walk around 128 thousand kilometres in their life time; that's more than three times around the earth. When walking, each time your heel lifts off the ground, it forces the toes to carry one half of your body weight.

If your feet were a car that had done a lot of kilometres, you would pay attention to warning signs, schedule regular tune-ups and get yourself a good mechanic!

My podiatry clinic, Alternative Foot Solutions in Manly, is the only podiatry clinic in New South Wales that specialises in Foot Mobilisation Therapy (FMT). My aim is to provide a medical solution to heal your aching body without pain, expensive surgery or orthotics, and therefore, improve the quality of your life for years to come.

Foot Mobilisation Therapy uses a gentle and painless hands-on technique to mobilise joints and improve the alignment of the feet and body. When a joint is not fully mobile, the surrounding joints take up the slack, creating extra stress all around.

Poor mobility in one area can cause pain and stress in other parts of the body. When combined with corrective exercises, FMT will fix the cause of foot, heel, ankle, leg, knee, hip and back pain. Alternative Foot Solutions provides a treatment program that has been developed over the years in consultation with my patients.

Hallux Abducto Varus, or 'bunions' as they are otherwise called, is one of the most common issues that we treat at Alternative Foot Solutions. The biggest misconception is that the only way to straighten the big toe is surgery.

This isn't true. We can reduce bunions effectively, and also comparatively cheaply, without causing you either undue pain, or forcing you to change your footwear or lifestyle.

Bunions are an all too common podiatry problem.

Foot pain from bunions affects over 30% of the Australian population. The bunion is defined as a swelling and misalignment at the point where the Hallux bone joins the Metatarsal, so essentially, it's where your big toe joins your mid-foot. What is conclusive is that bunions are caused by the misalignment in your foot, which in turn, affects the way that you stand and walk.

To correct your bunion long term, you need to address these underlying causes.

CHAPTER ONE

What is a Bunion?

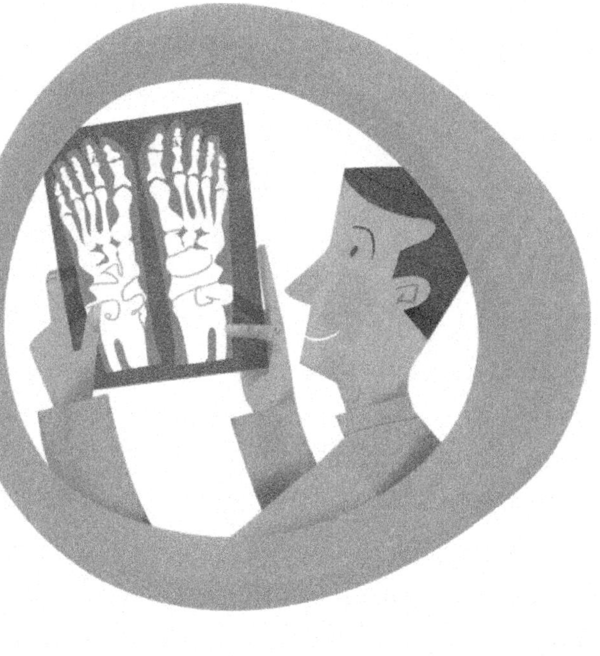

Bunions

A bunion is a broad term that describes the deformity of the Metatarsophalangeal Joint (MPTJ) or the big toe. The technical name is Hallux Abducto Valgus. The technical name is thus named, because a bunion is primarily a deviation of the big toe towards the centre of the foot and the lesser digits.

It is common for a bony growth to be associated with the misalignment that causes a bunion. Bunions are characterised by swelling and misalignment of the area where your big toe joins your mid-foot.

They are an all too common podiatry problem.

Foot pain from bunions affects over one in three Australians. According to doctors and most podiatrists, the only way to fix a bunion is surgery.

Many people remain unaware of the fact that here's a painless and natural way to effectively treat and correct your bunions, which doesn't require either expensive surgery or orthotics.

You can fix your bunion without surgery

Recent studies suggest that the prevalence of bunions in seniors within Australia could be as high as 70 percent.

Surgery to correct bunions is the fourth most common joint procedure, but unfortunately, surgery for bunions can result in complications, take significant healing time and cost thousands of dollars. It also affects mobility, and can also lead to extremely limited footwear options, especially for women.

Since a bunion is a deviation of the big toe towards the middle of the foot, if treatment is delayed, a bony growth causes a bump or an enlargement on the side and over the top of the big toe.

Given that there is a misalignment within the joint, bunions are usually, but not always painful, and they generally result in osteoarthritis within the big toe joint.

Accordingly, the best results for treatment are obtained when treatment is sought during the earlier development of a bunion.

Bunions are primarily caused by the alignment of your joints, the way that you stand and the way you walk. There is a hereditary link, so it's not uncommon for family members to share this condition.

Studies suggest that bunions can affect quality of life in a large number of cases. They are commonly associated with chafing in footwear, and are often a source of embarrassment due to the altered appearance of the feet.

Mobility can be limited and balance can be affected. Many people put off treatment because the area does not hurt. Unfortunately, by the time they do something about it, their only option is usually surgery.

There is a very effective, painless way to correct bunions that's been around for decades. The technique is foot mobilisation therapy (FMT). FMT is a gentle, hands-on technique that corrects the alignment of the foot and the bunion, and then uses exercises to strengthen the muscles around the joint to reinforce the position.

This technique is gentle, it involves minimal risk, and it does not limit footwear or activity. In fact, people are encouraged to continue their normal activities. The treatment actually corrects the underlying cause of the bunion in the first place, so the change is long-term.

Many people are unaware that this specialised technique exists.

Not many osteopaths or podiatrists practice this technique because it involves additional study.

Alternative Foot Solutions (AFS) is the only practice in NSW that specialises in foot mobilisation and the correction of bunions. The AFS clinic is located on the beaches in Manly, and practitioners Daniel and Lachlan, have over 13 years of experience in treating bunions through FMT.

If you are interested to find out more about this relatively unknown treatment for bunions, there are a number of resources at: *www.alternativefootsolutions.com.au*

Do You Have A Bunion And Think Surgery Is The Only Answer?

Do you have any of these Bunion Problems?

» Big Toe deviation
» Difficulty fitting into shoes
» Bone starting to form over the big toe
» A history of Bunions in the family
» Pain when you're walking

Surgery is not the Answer

If you're reading this book, it's likely that either you or a family member is suffering from a bunion. So, if you have contemplated surgery or orthotics to treat your bunion, or you're yet to see about it, we are offering our readers a free initial consultation so we can discuss whether or not our surgery-free option is the best option for your feet.

During our consultation, you can expect:

- An in-depth consultation about your bunion.
- A complete assessment to find the "cause" of your problem.
- An explanation of the underlying cause and how we fix your bunion.

Call us today on 02 89669300, and soon you could be walking towards pain-free walking in the shoes of your choice.

This a before and after X-ray, measuring the improvement of one of our patients after just the initial phase of treatment through foot mobilisation.

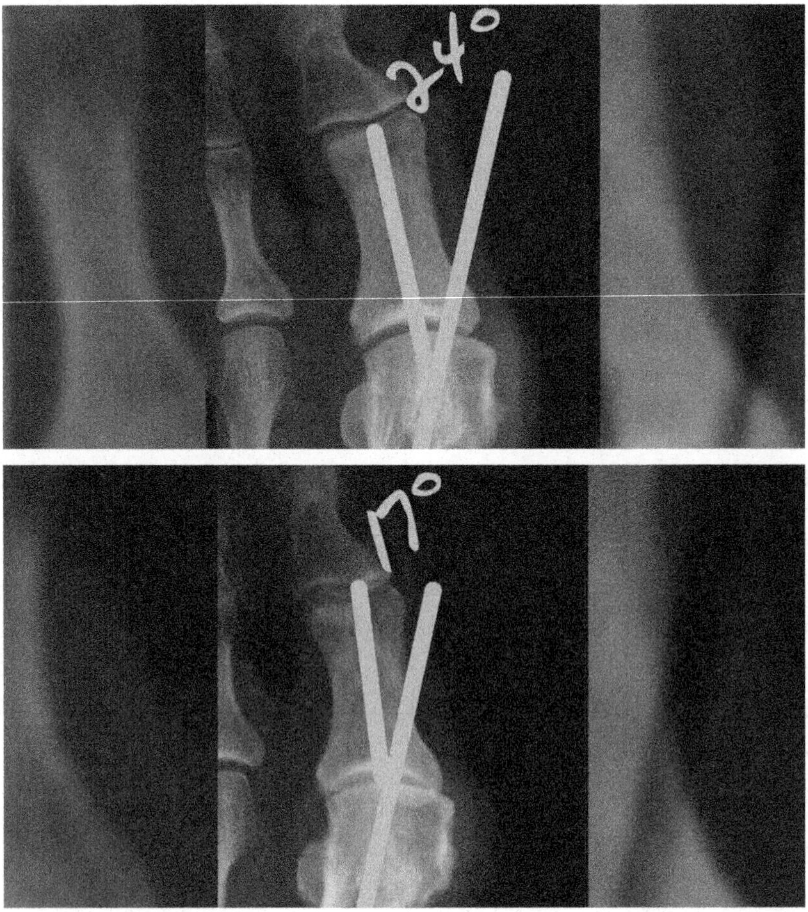

As you can see, the toe has straightened from 24 degrees to 17 degrees. The great news is that we would expect a complete straightening of her bunion; that is, a completely straight toe of only 15 degrees.

Still, there is a time and a place for surgery. The only time that someone would need to consider surgery though is if the bony callous growing out from a bunion needs to be cut off, but this would be in extreme cases only.

Most good quality surgeons are reluctant to consider this option unless the person is in crippling pain. For example, a line from one surgeon whom I consider among the best in his field is: “Come back and see me when you can’t walk”, which is akin to saying that patients should only consider this procedure in the event that there are no other viable options for treatment.

The need for surgery is rare, and it is indicated for extreme cases only. Surgery involves significant recovery time, it is expensive, and patients also lose function in the toe after the procedure.

Many post surgical patients report that they can’t exercise freely after surgery, and they never get back into the shoes they love.

Surgery should always be the last resort. In any case, you must remember that if surgery doesn’t go well or there is a complication, it usually affects the person’s quality of life, while this is not the scenario for foot mobilisation or other styles of conservative management.

CHAPTER TWO

What Causes a Bunion

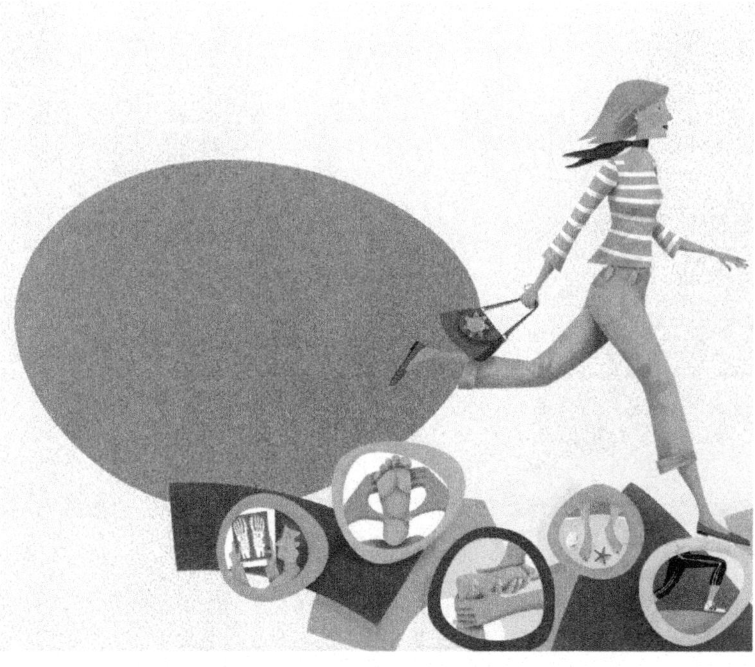

A bunion is primarily caused by the misalignment of your joints. This misalignment then affects the way that you stand and the way that you walk.

There are certain foot characteristics and walking patterns that are associated with bunions, which place extra stress on the big toe and push it out of alignment when someone stands and walks.

The force through your big toe joint exceeds two times your body weight when you walk, so if there is misalignment and the force isn't pushing the joint in the right direction, it's easy to see how someone gets a deviation in their big toe, which in turn, forms a bunion. If you add thousands of daily steps into the mix, it's easy to see how bunions can rapidly become worse!

Hereditary Factors

One of the most common things we hear at our clinic is: "I don't want Bunions like my Mother/Grandmother'. There is no doubt that there is a link between bunions and hereditary factors, which are biological traits that are passed down via genetics.

The traits that cause bunions that are passed down are related to misalignment in the lower limb; this misalignment will affect the force through the big toe when someone stands and walks, and can lead to a bunion.

The way a bunion forms and develops is the reason why we can straighten a bunion; we can improve the misalignment through the joints of the whole lower limb. The alignment of someone's feet will affect the way the muscles pull on the big toes and can further emphasise a bunion in someone's big toe.

Therefore, when were treat a bunion, we not only improve the alignment of the joints of the whole foot, we also strengthen the relevant muscles around the joint.

We generally find that the exercises we use as part of our treatment represent about 30 percent of the improvements we see.

Shoes

Tight shoes that are either too short in length or too tight through the toe box can contribute to bunions.

This problem usually applies more commonly to females, mainly because many women's shoes are cut away to give a more slimline and feminine appearance. Recent research suggests that tight footwear will definitely contribute to the development of any bunions that may already be in the process of developing.

Nevertheless, it would be unusual for tight footwear to be the only cause of the formation of a bunion.

Heels

Heels are not good for the muscular skeletal system, and they are blamed for being a leading underlying cause of bunions far more often than they should.

There is no doubt that the pressure that heels place directly on your big toe can accelerate a deviation of the big toe, and thus cause a bunion, but there usually has to be misalignment and other factors within the lower limb in order for a bunion to develop.

This point is further emphasised by the amount of bunions we assess, particularly when the patient reports that they've never worn heels!

Ballet and other dancing Activity

At our practice, we do attract quite a lot of dancers of all descriptions who suffer from a variety of foot conditions, with bunions being the most common. There is ongoing and significant debate in regards to whether participating in different forms of dance causes bunions.

In short, the answer to this question depends upon the type of movement; by far the most damaging form of dance to feet is ballet, and in particular, when adolescents transition to en pointe. Given the extreme nature of ballet, particularly in the advanced stages, you can see why ballet may increase the risk of a bunion.

I would definitely say that if someone has a genetic tendency and possesses the underlying predisposition that causes bunions, then pointe work from ballet will definitely accelerate this tendency.

For someone who is actively ballet dancing, we can usually do a lot to slow the process, improve the alignment and strengthen the relevant muscles, so that we can help to slow down, and in many cases, prevent further development of a bunion.

In terms of being able to straighten the toe, it is usually the case that this is difficult while that person is still doing pointe work. In regards to other forms of dance and their propensity to cause bunions, it once again really depends on whether the individual has the misalignment and the tendencies that facilitate bunions in the first place.

Usually a contributing factor for dancers presenting to us for treatment is that they cannot wear supportive or ideal footwear while whilst engaging this activity. As a result, if the individual does suffer with significant misalignment of the lower limb, then this will increase the negative forces on the big toe joint, and in some cases, cause damage in the form of a bunion.

So, if you do partake in a form of dancing, I wouldn't suggest giving it up just because your Mum or someone in your family has a bunion. I would though suggest you get assessed by someone who knows how to address the underlying cause of a bunion so that you can avoid the issue.

Too Much activity, such as long distance running

Running is definitely not a cause of bunions and being active isn't a cause of bunions either, provided you don't have the genetic and bio-mechanical tendencies to develop bunions. The reality is though that when you exercise for longer periods, your body will fatigue.

As a consequence of this fatigue, your leg misalignment increases, because the muscles supporting your joints become fatigued, and the outcome of this is that they cannot maintain their position any longer.

It is when you are fatigued that you are at greatest risk of injury or damage, because you cannot maintain a good postural position. The implication of bodily fatigue during running is that you should try to to avoid maintaining the same pace throughout the work-out.

Instead, exercise intervals are particularly good to combat fatigue, or alternatively, HIIT (High intensity interval training), because your body can continue to maintain good posture while still getting a good workout. It has also been shown that it is much better for your joints in general.

When can bunions start?

Bunions can start as early as eleven-years-old in girls, and a little older in boys. Consequently, we treat a lot of adolescents, which allows us the ability to assist these patients in the avoidance of future issues.

However, there are no hard and fast rules, because there are a number of factors that influence when a bunion will either develop or progress. Furthermore, foot alignment can change over the course of someone's life, and consequently, this can affect the big toe, and in turn, can lead to the development of a bunion.

We know that the incidence of bunions increases dramatically after the age of 65, but there are other factors that influence the development of a bunion. For example, pregnancy is a common time when women's feet change due to the hormonal impact on the connective tissues in the feet.

The Top Two Underlining Causes of Foot Problems and how to fix them for good!

Unless it's an acute incident (i.e. falling and hurting yourself), most people's foot problems that we see at Alternative Foot Solutions are chronic, and their foot issues happen over a period of time, and bit by bit.

Most people don't realise that this is the case, and in their defence, some contemporary research suggests that people might only feel the most recent deterioration in their feet (approximately 7% of the overall foot pathology).

In other words, people don't begin to feel most of the damage until it's too late.

The damage or inflammation that leads to the pain is usually caused by two main factors, or it usually has two main underlying causes.

We find that a number of our patients who attend our clinic are frustrated that no-one has either discussed their problem or worked out a plan to address the underlying causes of their foot problems.

Underlying cause 1- Misalignment or Subluxation

The first underlying cause of foot problems is misalignment or subluxation, which essentially means that if your joints are out of alignment, this misalignment will affect the way that you stand or walk.

This, in turn, will place your joints, connective tissues and soft tissues under increased load, and therefore, your body has to compensate. Your body's attempt to compensate will lead to micro-tears, and these micro-tears will bleed and become inflamed. This eventually leads to pain.

Underlying case 2- Muscle Weakness in Arch and Big Toe

If the muscles in the arch and big toe function poorly or are weak, they will contribute to a bunion forming. Of course, the function of these muscles is heavily affected by the alignment or misalignment of your joints. The great thing about this is that it's relatively easy to build up these muscles if you know how.

We know that in bunion correction that the exercises account for 30 % of the improvement or correction we see when treating patients.

The downside is that the results in terms of correcting your bunion or preventing a bunion are extremely limited if you don't receive foot mobilisation treatment at the same time. If you don't get the alignment of your joints corrected via foot mobilisation, you won't correct a bunion and you won't be able to stop one.

We have people contact us all the time saying they did their exercises but it didn't stop or fix their bunion. I then ask them whether they attended our clinic, and the answer is, "No". I reply that, for two reasons, I'm not shocked by their response:

» The key underlying causes, i.e., the misalignment, hasn't been treated;
» The main reason that most of our patients stick to the exercises is that they are coming to see us and we keep the patient accountable. Keep in mind, the exercises only take a few minutes per day, but people do their exercises, particularly if they know we will be following up with them.

How to Fix This Forever!

In my experience, if you fix this misalignment, then you address the underlying cause. In fixing the alignment, you stop the process and allow the body to heal itself naturally, and in doing so, the body stays better forever.

The way we do this at Alternative Foot Solutions is by gently guiding the joints back into their best position through a hands-on technique and then supporting this change with exercises that you can do while you clean your teeth.

We believe it's important to address the underlying cause naturally, and without resorting to a short-term band-aid solution.

CHAPTER THREE

Why You Should Fix a Bunion and Myths about Bunions

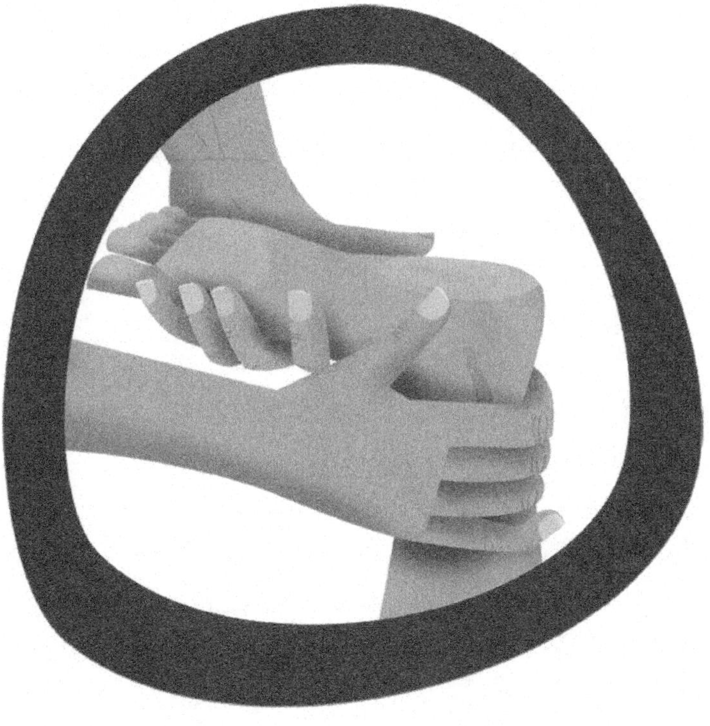

Reasons to fix a bunion NOW!

The fact is, it's only going to get worse.

Generally, once the big toe starts to deviate, it will generally continue to deviate more significantly. I'm not in the business of fear mongering, and I am always happy to be proven wrong, but unfortunately in this case the bunion is not likely to go away, without intervention.

The reason that it will keep deviating is because, unfortunately, the reasons bunions develop in the first place won't suddenly change. That is, you won't all of a sudden start to walk and stand differently. So with each passing step, you will place increasing pressure and weight on the big toe joint, thereby causing increased deviation and damage.

Once the deviation gets to a certain point, a few things will happen. The first is that when the bone is under stress, it typically lays down more bone. The problem with laying down more bone is the extra bone that creates the big lump on the side of the foot; this is lump is irreversible, and the only way to fix it is surgery.

It can be cut off, which will be discussed in greater depth later in this chapter.

The other issue is that the excessive negative forces on the big toe will start to wear the joint out, causing degenerative change. This degenerative change generally leads to the painful condition of osteoarthritis. This condition affects people's quality of life. We can work with this condition, but it's not an ideal situation.

The other issue is that if you delay having treatment, you are limiting your options.

When we assess a bunion, we measure in degrees how much it has deviated from anatomically straight toes, which invariably measure between 12-15 degrees.

If you delay treatment for long enough, then your options become severely limited. I strongly suggest that if you have a bunion, whether or not it hurts, that you get it assessed as soon as possible.

Surgery will be your only option if you leave it long enough. So, when it comes to bunions, there are some cases where we can fix the bunion with conservative management, but in extreme cases, there is a time and a place for surgery.

The only other time that surgery would be indicated is if you have an excessive amount of bone jutting out of the side of your toe. Nonetheless, getting the bony callous removed as opposed to straightening the toe is a very different surgery, with far less involved.

When it comes to the surgery people don't usually take into account what's involved and what the long term outcomes will be. I'm the first to admit that there are some patients who have bunions that are too far gone. We cannot fix every bunion, but regardless, surgery should always be last resort.

Surgery

If conservative measures do not work for you and you continue to experience pain that impacts your daily activities, then you may require surgery. Nevertheless, bunion surgery should always be a last resort, and it's important to be realistic in regards to your expectations about what surgery will achieve.

Furthermore, you will be required to remain off your foot for at least six to 12 weeks after the surgery. Complete recovery can take a year or even longer, depending on the procedure.

As with any surgery, you will need to ensure that the physician who is performing the surgery is experienced in performing the particular operation you've decided to undergo.

The chief objective of the surgery is to relieve pain and to restore normal function via eliminating the bony protuberance at the side of the foot and realigning the joint, which includes, tendons, ligaments, and nerves).

There are more than 100 surgical procedures for bunion correction, but few of them have been evaluated or compared in controlled trials.

Before a decision is made in regards to the type of surgery is best for your situation, the surgeon will take X-rays and measurements that help classify the bunion as either mild, moderate, or severe.

Your age, activity level, health, and the strength of your bones and connective tissue are also factors that are taken into account to guide the decision about the best type of surgery for you. The more severe the bunion, the more complicated and potentially risky the surgery.

For only mild cases, the physician will probably perform a procedure called a bunionectomy, which involves shaving off the enlarged portion of the bone, and then realigning the muscles, tendons, and ligaments. For moderate deformities, it may be necessary to cut the bone close to the metatarsal head in order to place it back into its correct position.

To correct severe bunions, the physician will need to make a cut at the base of the metatarsal bone, rotate the bone, and then attach it in place with pins or screws. The process of cutting and repositioning the bones is called an osteotomy.

These different types of surgical procedures can be performed under local, general, or spinal anesthesia on an outpatient basis within a hospital setting, at a surgical center, or at a doctor's surgery. The procedure is usually carried out by an orthopedic, podiatric, or other specialist foot surgeon.

Downsides to surgery

Risk

There is always a risk with any surgery; if it doesn't go well, it will impact the quality of a person's life longer term.

Alternatively, if conservative management doesn't work, then it may certainly be a waste of time and money, but it would be extremely rare for it to cause long term damage.

Another major disadvantage of surgery is that surgery will lead to an overall decrease in activity. For instance, the common feedback we get form people is that after bunion surgery, they can't walk as far or as easily, particularly if the surgery involved straightening of the toe and pinning the area.

In addition, the recovery from surgery is usually far longer than people usually realise and plan for. Generally speaking, it's six weeks in a boot, however it's not unusual for people to report swelling for 12 to 18 months after the procedure.

The other issue that is particularly relevant to women is that once the toe has been pinned, the amount of flexion in the toe can be limited, and this is particularly problematic for women who wish to wear heels again.

Complication rates of surgery for bunions across a number of studies range from 10% to 55%. The most common complication is recurrence of the bunion, which has been reported in as many as 16% of cases.

This complication can occur when only the bony prominence at the side of the toe is shaved off but the underlying flexion problem that caused the issue isn't corrected.

In some cases of surgery, the cut bone heals too slowly, and in rarer cases, it doesn't come back together at all. This condition, called nonunion, which will require additional surgery. Among additional complications to surgery are irritation from the pins and screws that are used to hold the bone together, in addition to extensive scarring or stiffness.

The swelling that is usually quite prominent after surgery tends to ease within two months, but on some occasions, it can last for six months or longer. While nerve damage and ongoing pain are rare, they still occur, which serve to lengthen recovery time. In some cases, additional surgery may be required for nerve damage and persistent pain.

COMMON MYTHS ABOUT BUNIONS

5 Bunion Myths

Myth # 1 The only treatment for bunions is surgery.

This is not true. At Alternative Foot Solutions, we commonly treat bunions. In most cases, we can correct the underlying deviation of the big toe without surgery, without change of footwear, and without orthotics.

Myth # 2 If it doesn't hurt, it's not a problem so I don't need to treat it.

This is not true. The joint is out of alignment, which causes wear and tear to the joint every time you walk or run. Eventually, the joint will wear out (much faster than you think!) and then you won't be able to do the things you love, like wear heels or fashionable shoes, run, or in many cases, walk freely without pain. The other issue is that when your big toe joint does wear out, it will take a toll on other joints in your body—right up to your neck!

Myth # 3 My doctor doesn't know about conservative management for bunions, so it can't work.

General practitioners cannot know about every treatment available for every condition. Patients who ask their local doctor about treatments for their bunions are often referred to a surgeon, but surgery should always be the last resort for bunions.

The great thing about conservative management is that it has no long-term ramifications, which surgery might have. Also, it involves much lower costs, and it exerts no negative impact on your quality of life. Most importantly, it works and we can measure our results.

As specialists in this area, we can offer a number of conservative management approaches to pursue before you consider surgery. In most cases, if you come to see us, you will never need to see the surgeon.

Myth # 4 Treatment will mean changing my footwear to "nanna" shoes.

At Alternative Foot Solutions, we are able to correct bunions without changing footwear and without orthotics. We do it consistently by gently mobilising the misalignment in your feet and strengthening the relevant muscles around the joint.

Myth # 5 My bunion isn't big enough to worry about.

The earlier we treat potential bunions, the better the outcome. The pattern that causes bunions is hereditary, and we have treated 12-year-old children to prevent bunions getting worse.

If you have any sign of a bunion, or if you have a family history of bunions, make an appointment as soon as possible.

At Alternative Foot Solutions, we believe in the earliest possible prevention (if possible). If you have a loved one with a bunion, whether it be advanced or just beginning, the sooner it's treated, the less it will cost, the less treatment it will take, and the better the outcome.

Just give us a call on 02 89669300 or visit our website at www.alternativefootsolutions.com.au and leave your details.

CHAPTER FOUR

Case Studies

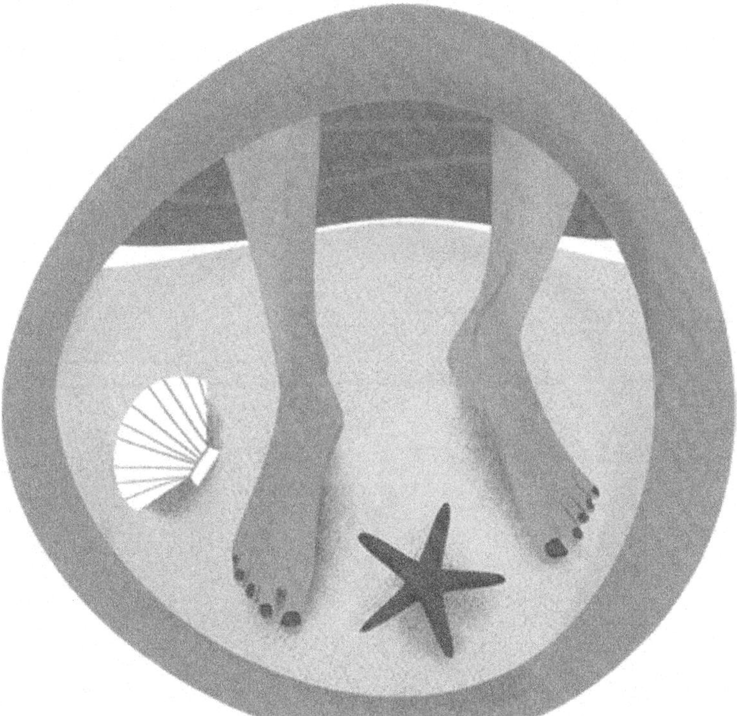

The case studies contained in Chapter 4 have been shared in order to showcase how effective our methods can be. In particular, our case studies illustrate that the treatments are relatively non-invasive, and also, that they work relatively fast.

Make sure you read this section of the book: In this section, we demonstrate how we carry out our treatments, exactly what is involved with each phase of treatment, and also, we will demonstrate via each of these cases what you can expect when you come to access our service. We've even included before and after X-rays to demonstrate the toe straightening process!

Do you have a bunion and think that your only option is surgery?

Are you worried that your bunion will just get worse?

Does someone in you family have bunions?

At Alternative Foot Solutions, we are the only clinic in NSW that can straighten your bunion naturally, and we believe you shouldn't have to resort to surgery or give up the shoes you love.

We do this through a method called Foot Mobilisation Therapy. This treatment gently corrects the alignment of your foot and big toe naturally and painlessly.

About 60 % of the patients we treat attend our clinic in regard to bunion correction. This is due to the fact that we are the only clinic in NSW that provides this unique approach to treating bunions naturally.

For those who don't know what a bunion is, its where there's a deviation of the big toe. We can actually correct this alignment and straighten the big toe, thereby avoiding long-term issues and painful, not to mention, expensive surgery.

We are very proud of our success dealing with bunions, and here are some before and after X-rays measuring the results over our treatment process.

If you don't think there's any hope for fixing your bunion without surgery, you have to read this!

Foot pain from bunions is prevalent in over 1 in 3 Australians.

The biggest misconception is that surgery is the only way to straighten the big toe. Not true. We can reduce bunions effectively—and comparatively cheaply, without causing pain or a change in footwear or lifestyle. Because are the only clinic that can naturally straighten your big toes, we are accustomed to skepticism. Nevertheless, we can give you hard proof (before and after X-rays) that we can straighten bunions.

The first X-ray is of a lady we treated for painful bunions, and she also suffered from osteoarthritis. She attended our clinic because her feet were very painful and she couldn't wear any fashionable shoes. We sent her for X-rays, and below was the result. The ideal reading for a straight big to is 12 to 15 degrees. I'm sure you agree we had some work to do.

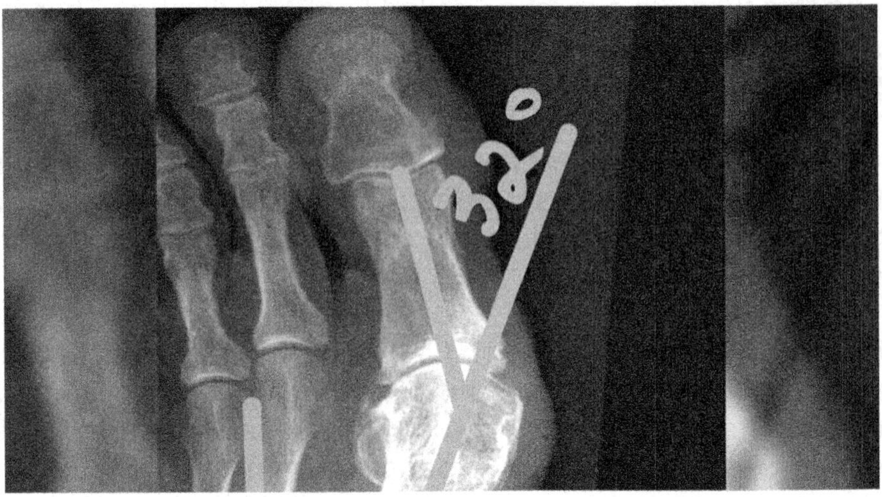

So after the initial phase of her corrective treatment, we X-rayed her again to measure the results. I'm happy to report that she had a seven degree reduction. Keep in mind that this is only after the initial correction phase of the treatment. Better still, there's no more pain.

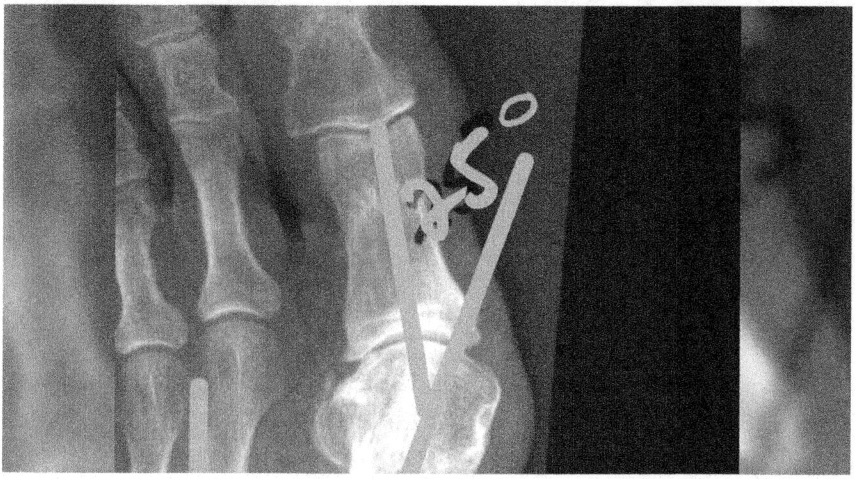

This is a before X-ray of a bunion that we recently corrected for one of our female patients who is 61 years young. Her name is Kay. Kay wanted to keep dancing and active, but also wear fashionable shoes. Kay has a sister who had had surgery which had not gone very well, so Kay was desperate to avoid surgery.

Accordingly, we sent for an X-ray to measure the misalignment, and we got a reading of 28 degrees, which we can see here. The ideal reading for a big toe is between 12-15 degrees, so we had some work to do.

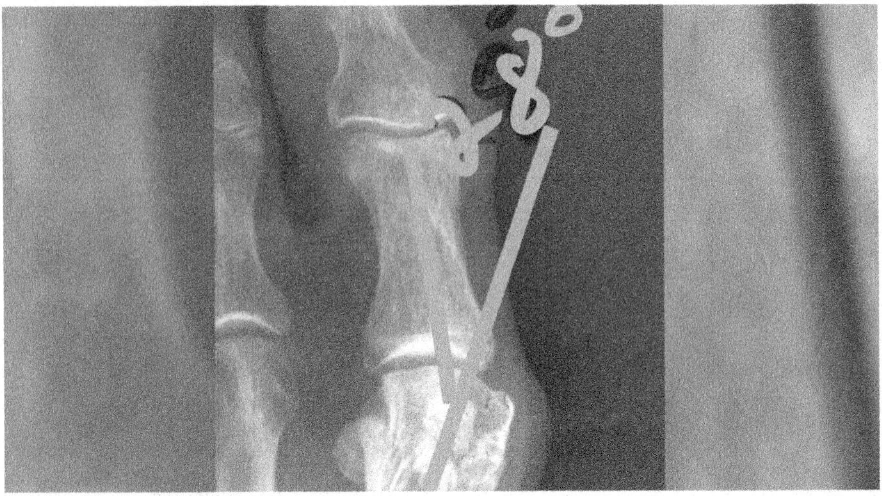

Her after X-ray is below. This was taken after the initial phase of treatment, and the improvement is remarkable considering she didn't have to stop doing anything, and she kept wearing the shoes she loved. Her deviation was down to 18 degrees.

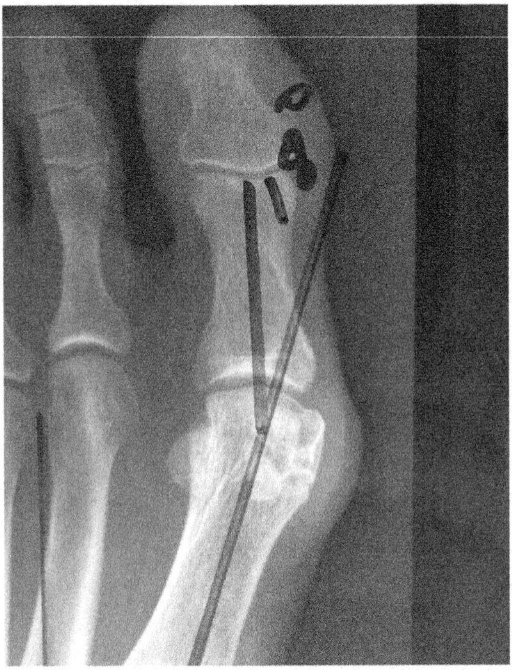

Here is another example of a bunion were we took a before and after X-ray. This time, the patient was a female in her late fifties.

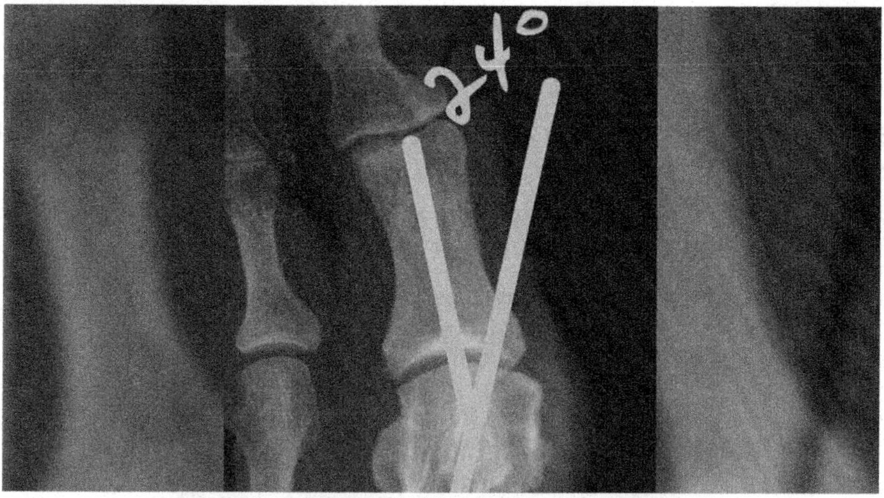

Once again, a great result was achieved after the initial corrective phase of the treatment, and there were only two degrees to go until we achieved a straight toe. This is a great result, especially considering the treatment is a gentle, hands-on technique that doesn't hurt.

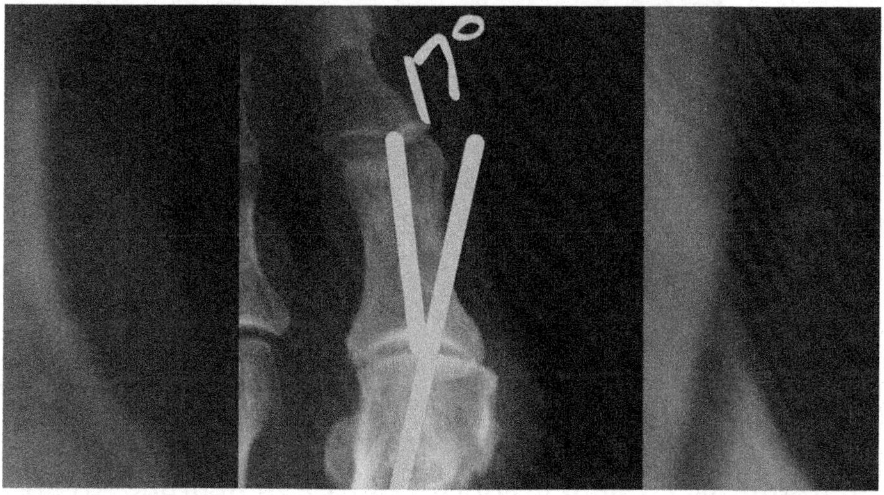

We have successfully treated thousands of bunions between us at Alternative Foot Solutions and believe that there is a better

alternative to surgery or constant pain due to a bunion.
We feel the sooner the bunion is treated, the better the long-term result.

Here are some more before and after x-rays of patients that are well on their way to correcting their bunion after x-ray were taken after only a few months of treatment the great news is that the best is yet to come and we would expect their bunion to keep correcting to the point where is anatomically straight.

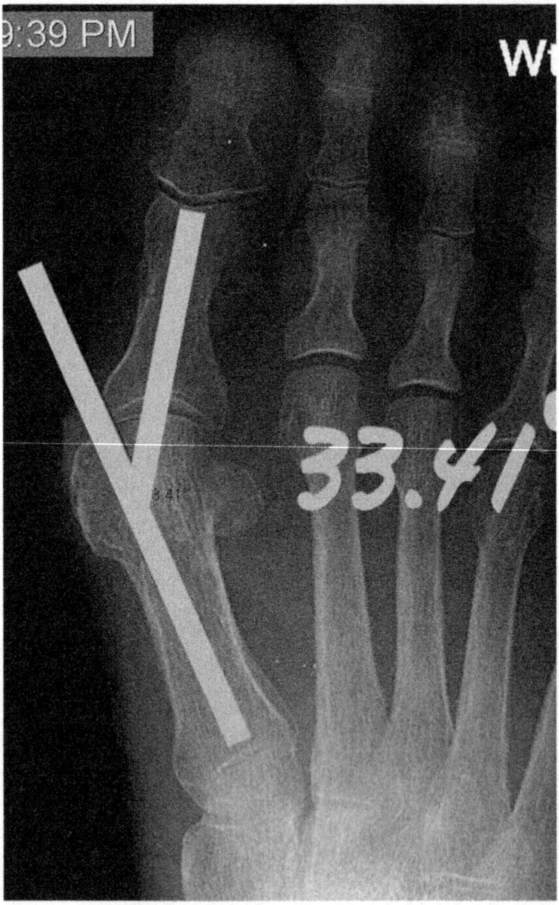

So anatomically straight is considered 12-15 degrees. So above is a before x-ray from a female patient in her mid-sixties that had a mild degenerative change with significant misalignment in her big toe at 33.4 degrees.

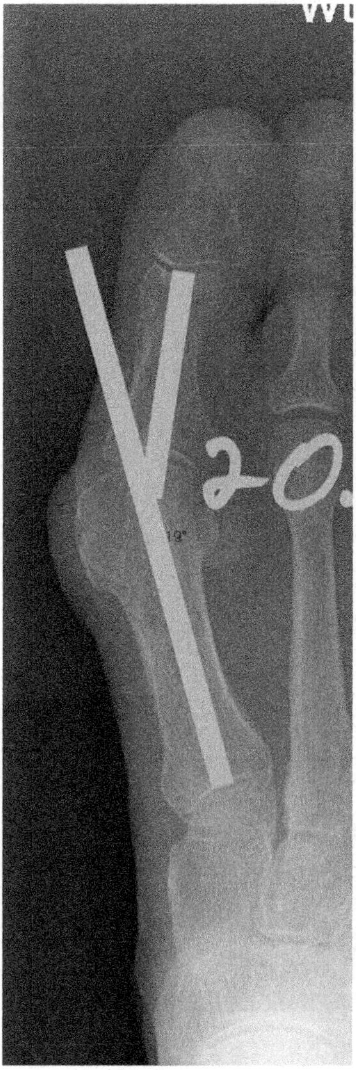

After a few months we x-rayed and saw over a 13 degree improvement the great news is that we would expect the toe to be straight. Not to mention no pain!

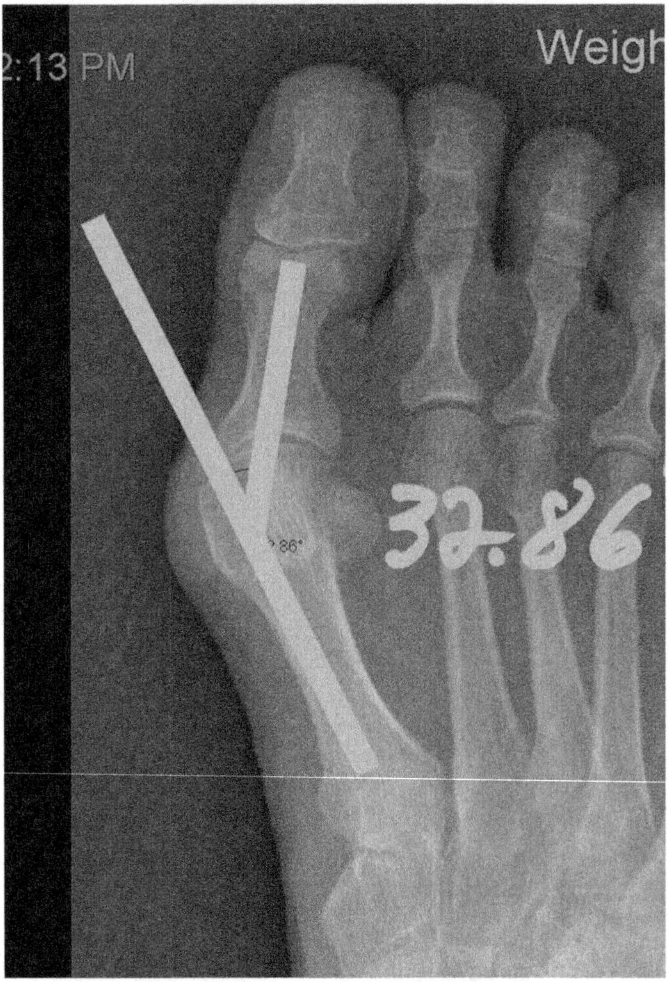

Our next x-ray belongs to a female patient in her 50's and she was 32.86 degrees when we met. She wasn't getting any pain but wanted to avoid surgery.

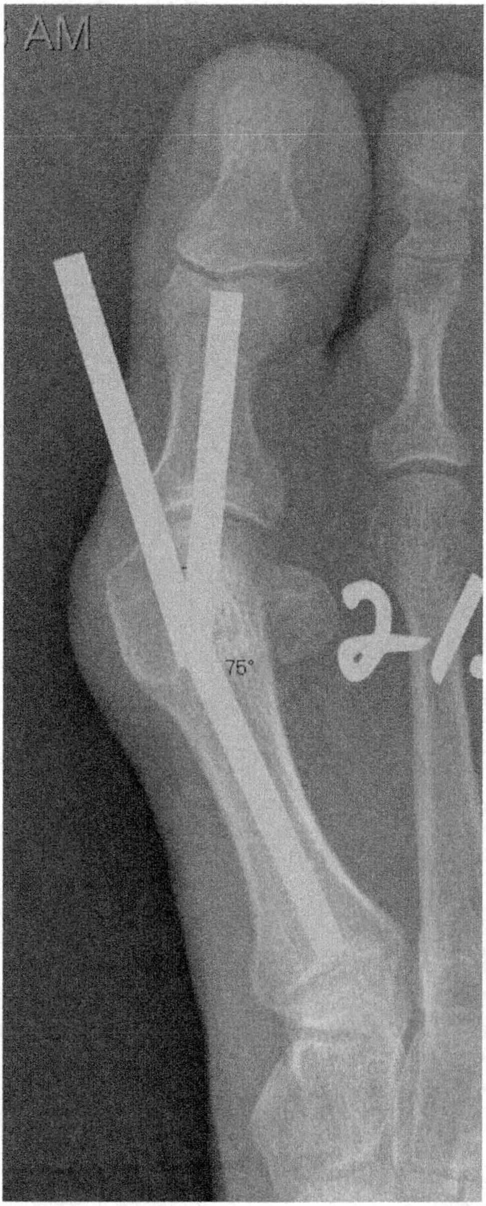

After an initial course of treatment we x-rayed and she was down to 21 degrees in just a number of weeks. We would expect her toe to keep straightening until it gets to 15 deg.

The next x-ray we see was another patient that was determined not to end up having surgery she came to see us and we x-rayed and found a deviation of the bunion of 26 degrees.

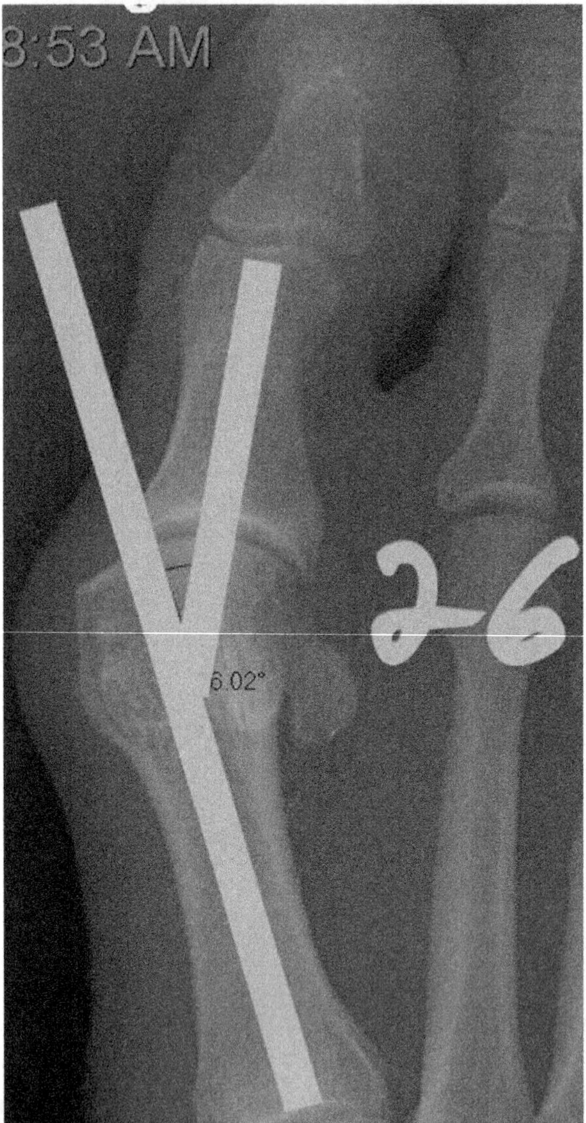

After the first phase of treatment were x-rayed and had a change down to 15 degrees which is anatomically straight. A great result and no need for surgery.

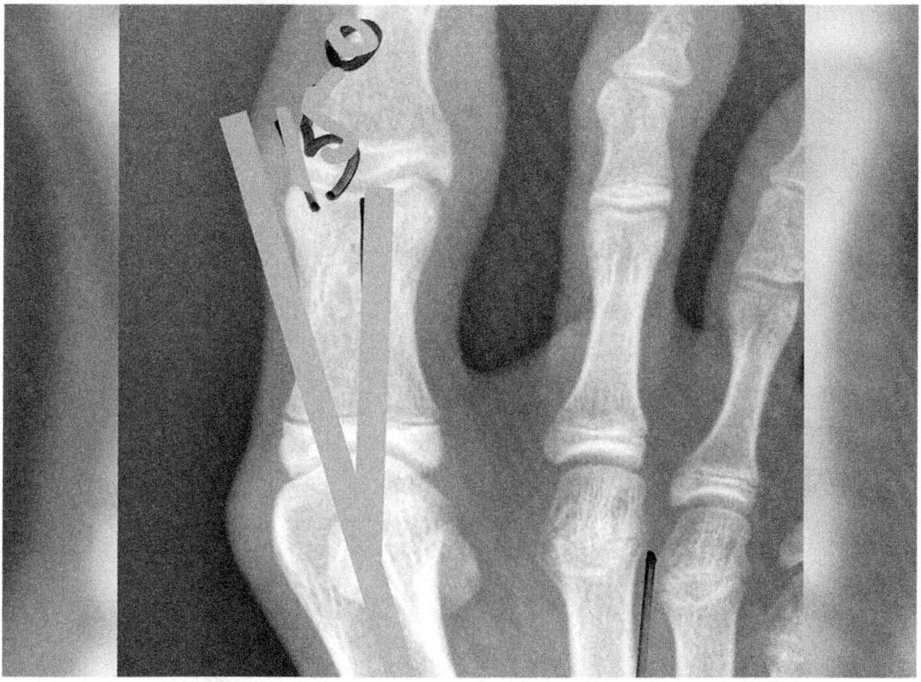

Our next x-ray the patient was well into her 70's and had osteoarthritis in the big toe and had significant amounts of pain. Her bunion was 30.45 degrees.

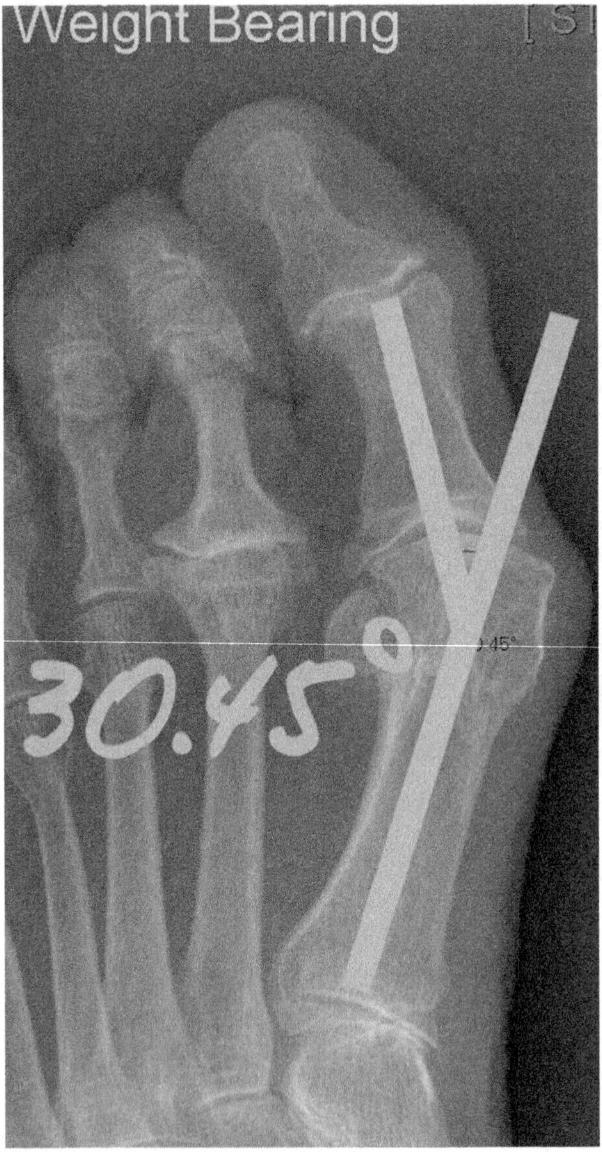

So we reduced the pain this patient was getting not to mention reduced her bunion angle down to 23.35 degrees. Despite OA being present we still got a great result, reduced pain and straightened the toe. This shows that you can straighten a bunion no matter what the age.

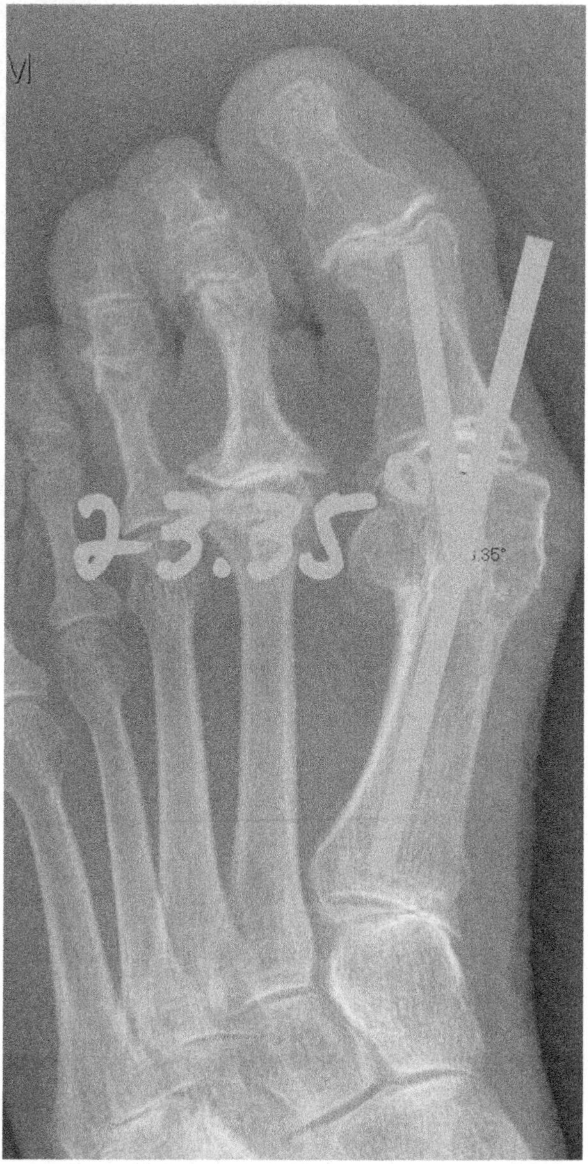

Here we see a younger patient's foot with a very developed bunion for his age at 27 degrees.

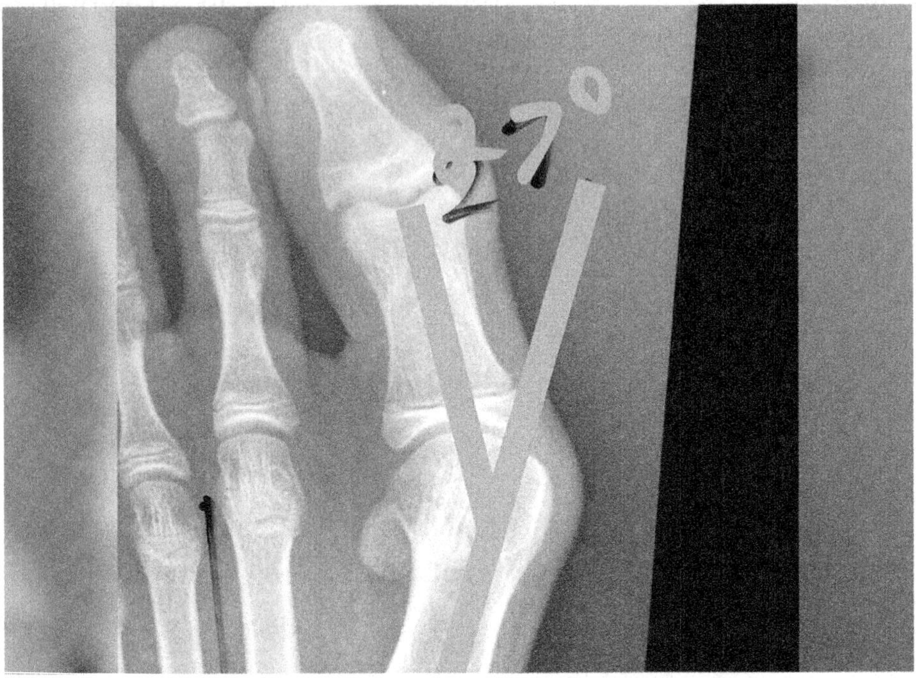

After a couple of month's (a month's or some months?) treatment we x-rayed and it was 14 degrees completely straight!

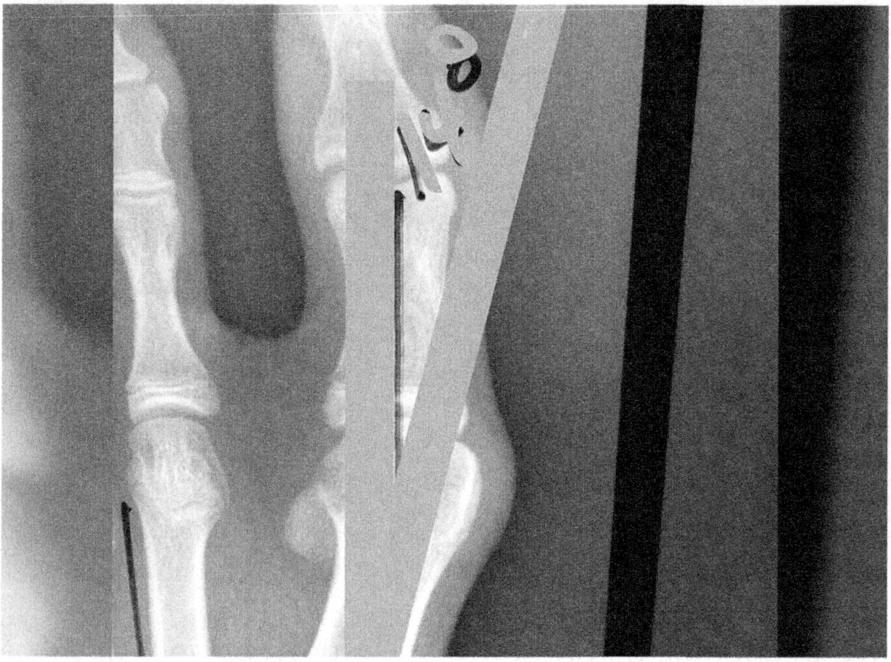

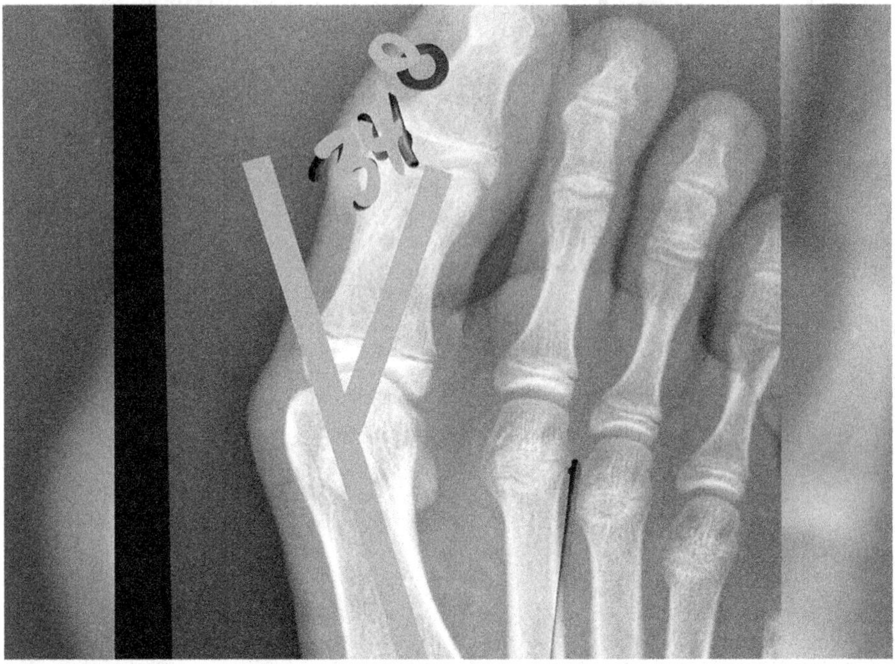

Above is another before x-ray at 34 degrees very advanced bunion.

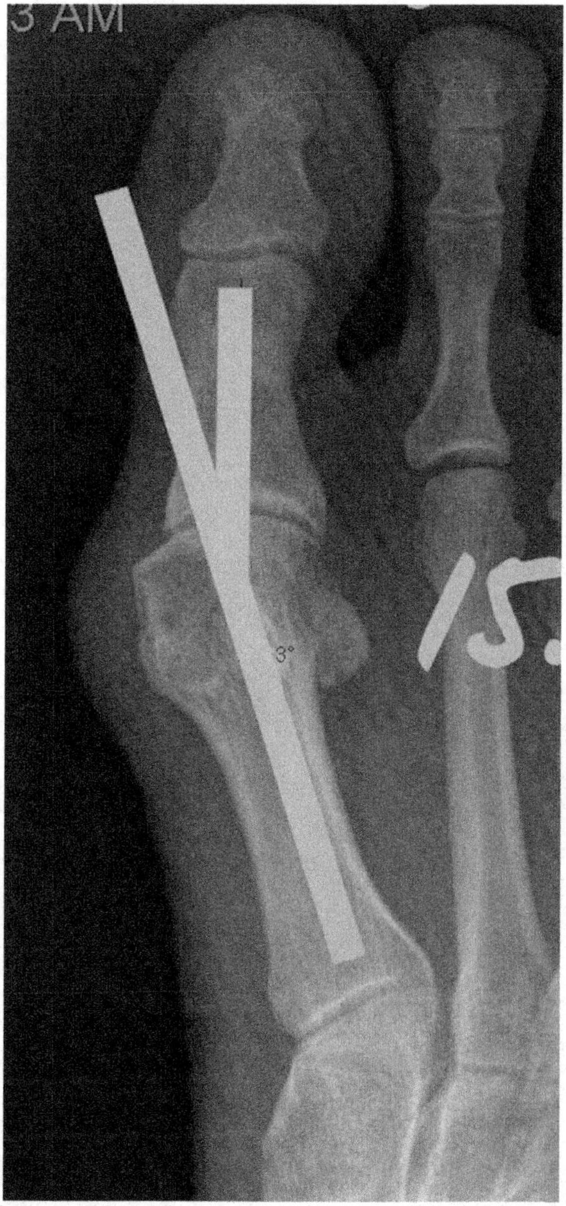

Above is the after a huge change from 34 degrees down to 15 degrees anatomically straight.

Another advanced bunion at 28 degrees.

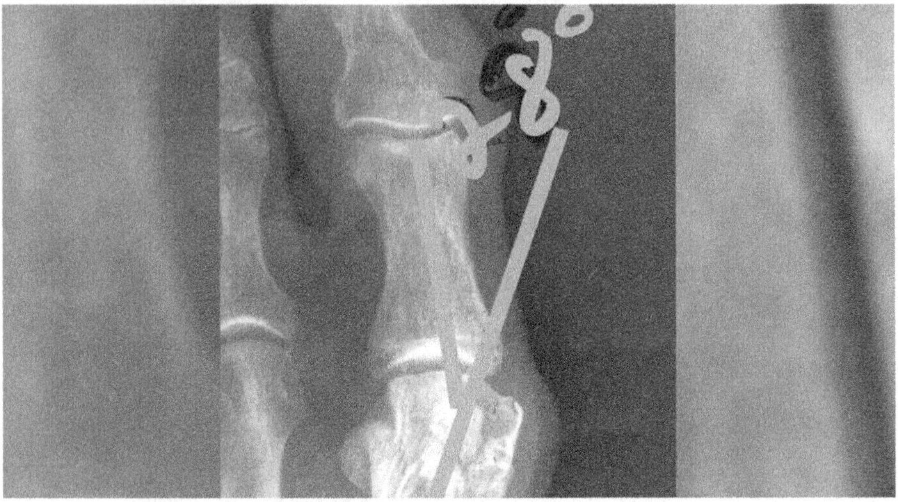

After is 20 degrees the great news is the best is yet to come we expect this to be 15 degrees in no time.

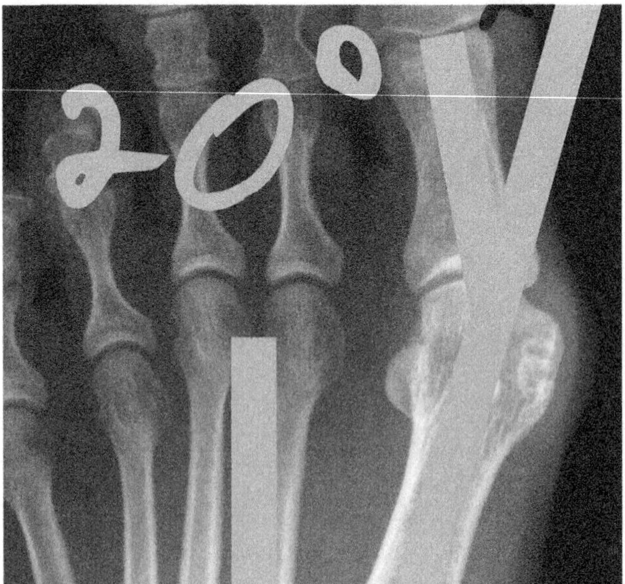

Linda's Case

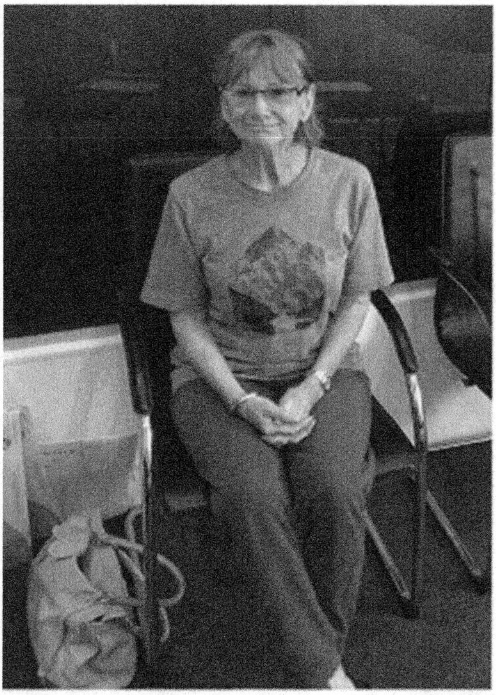

Meet Linda, aged 61. Linda is a patient with a classic case of bunions.

Linda had moderate bunions bilaterally; her big toe is turned inwards on both feet. She had endured foot pain for years, adjusting her footwear to accommodate the excessive deviation. Linda's case was complicated by osteoarthritis in her big toe joint, which is not uncommon in older patients.

We routinely incorporate patients' goals into our medical assessments. In Linda's case, her goal was to avoid painful and expensive surgery, as well as to remain active.

Linda was pleasantly surprised when we told her that we could actually straighten the big toe and reduce her bunions without her having to sacrifice high heels or reduce her general activity. Linda was already wearing sensible footwear on most occasions, but she wanted the option to wear heels should she choose to in future.

Following our initial assessment, which included an X-ray, we decided upon course of foot mobilisation podiatry in conjunction with strengthening exercises.

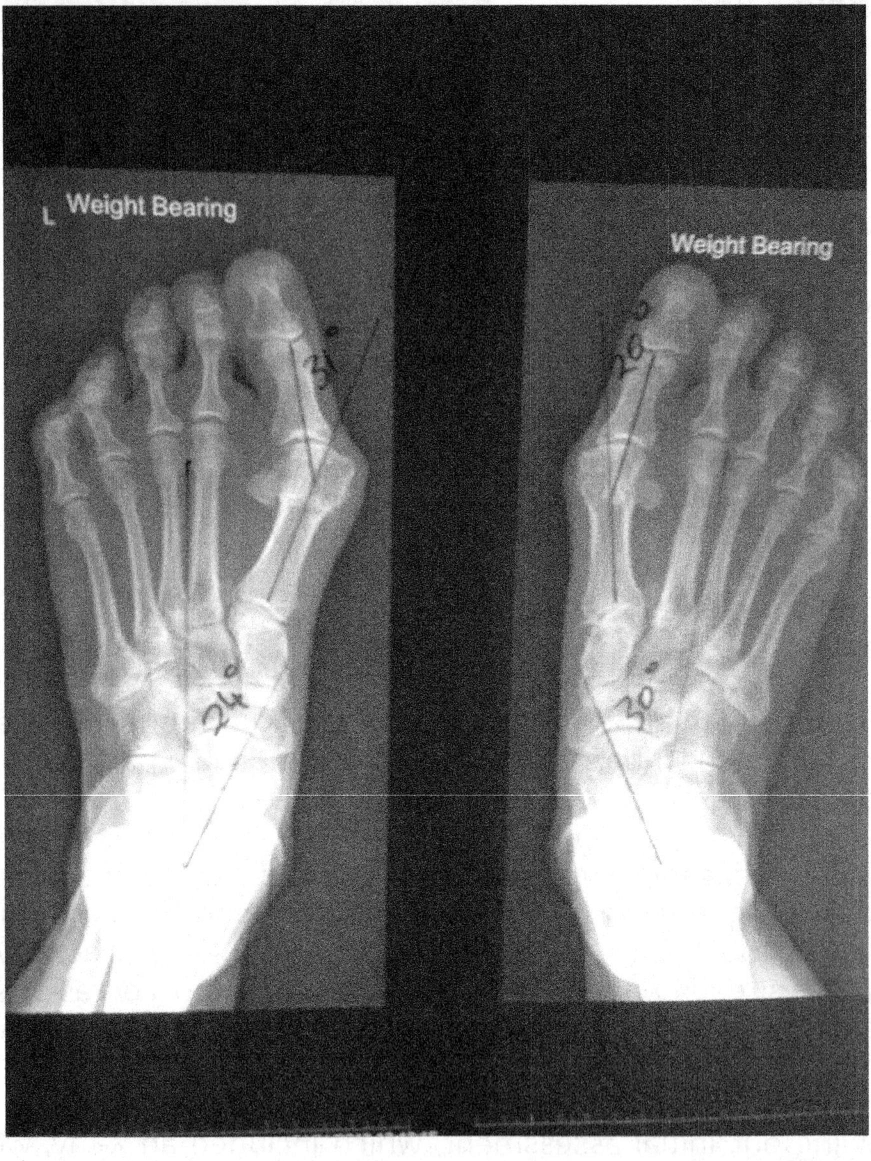

Our podiatry treatment showed improvement within just a month.

To her credit, Linda participated enthusiastically in the appointments and the exercises. We noticed a reduction in her bunions within four weeks of commencing treatment.

During that time, Linda commented that she could see her big toe straightening.

Results

On measuring the difference between the angles of deviation before and after treatment, we found that we had straightened the left toe by 7 degrees and the right by 8 degrees. The great news is that with minimal ongoing treatment, we will be able to further straighten the bunion until there is no deviation whatsoever. This magnitude of improvement only took three months, and the best is yet to come.

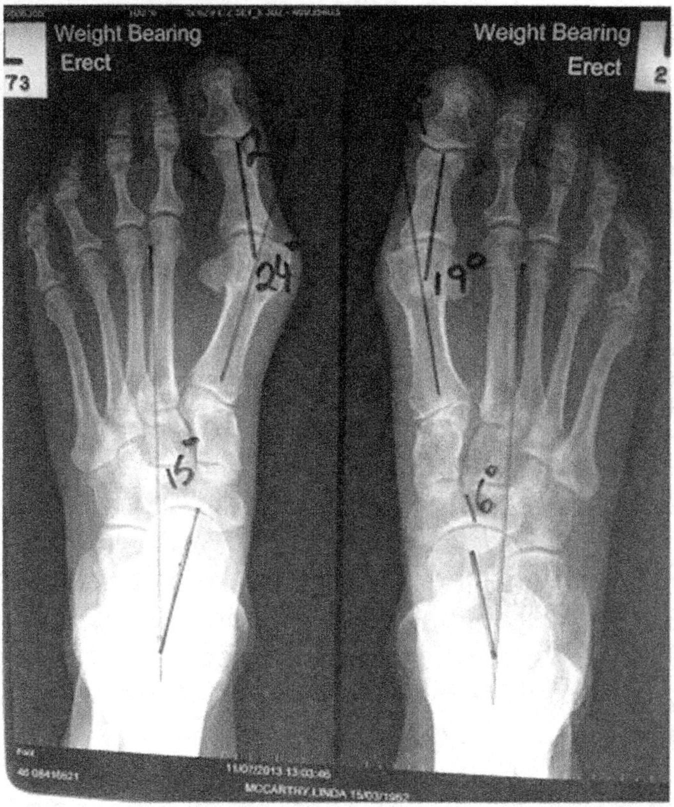

Well done to Linda! There was no need for expensive surgery, or for a change to her footwear!

Pam's Case

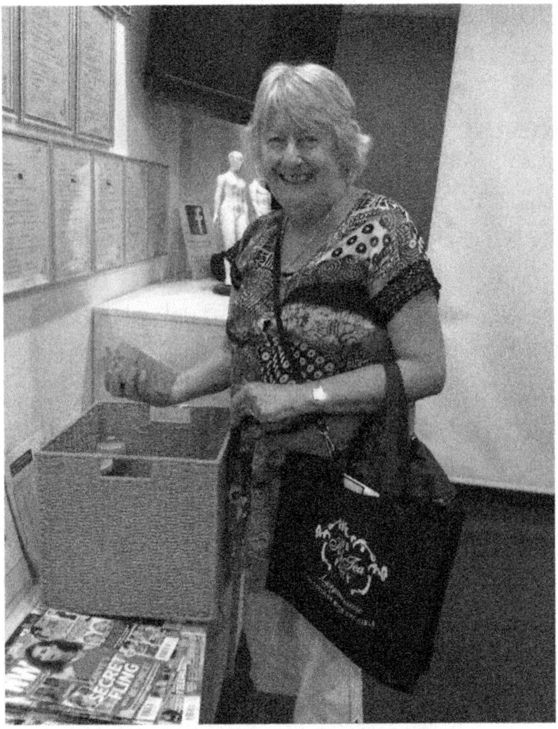

As Pam's case illustrates, you can fix your bunions naturally, even if most doctors think that surgery is your only option! I want to introduce you to Pam, a patient with a classic case of bunions.

Pam (aged 65) had moderate bunions bilaterally (the big toe turned inwards), and she had endured foot pain for many years. Furthermore, she had become accustomed to adjusting her footwear to accommodate the excessive deviation. Pam was referred to us by her sister.

Pam was pleasantly surprised to hear that we could actually straighten the big toe and reduce her bunions, without affecting her family commitments, in particular, her child-minding duties.

After establishing Pam's personal goals, we medically assessed her case during our initial consultation, which included an X-ray. This was Pam's initial X-ray. As you can see below, her initial X-ray confirmed a bunion angle of 25 degrees, whereas the ideal angle is 12-15 degrees.

We decided on a course of foot mobilisation podiatry in conjunction with strengthening exercises. I should also mention at this stage Pam was living in the Southerland Shire but since we are the only clinic in New South Wales that corrects bunions naturally, she was happy to catch the ferry over to our clinic. The treatment yielded improvement in Pam's bunions within just a month.

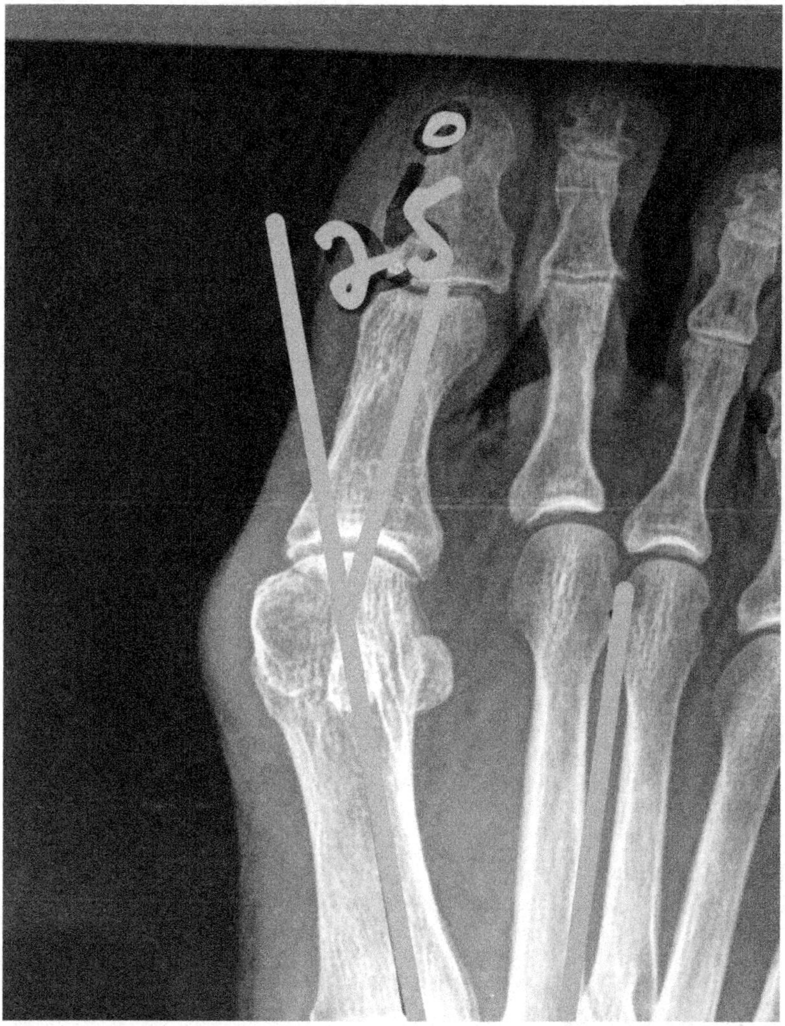

To her credit, Pam was enthusiastic about the appointments and the exercises. We noticed a reduction in her bunions within just four weeks of commencing treatment. During that time, Pam commented that she could see her big toe straightening.

In Pam's case, the four weeks were the most intense aspect of the treatment, with a reduction in the frequency of her visits after that.

As we do with all our bunion corrections, we sent Pam for a follow-up X-ray to measure her results. Pam's bunions had reduced to just 19 degrees, which is a huge improvement.

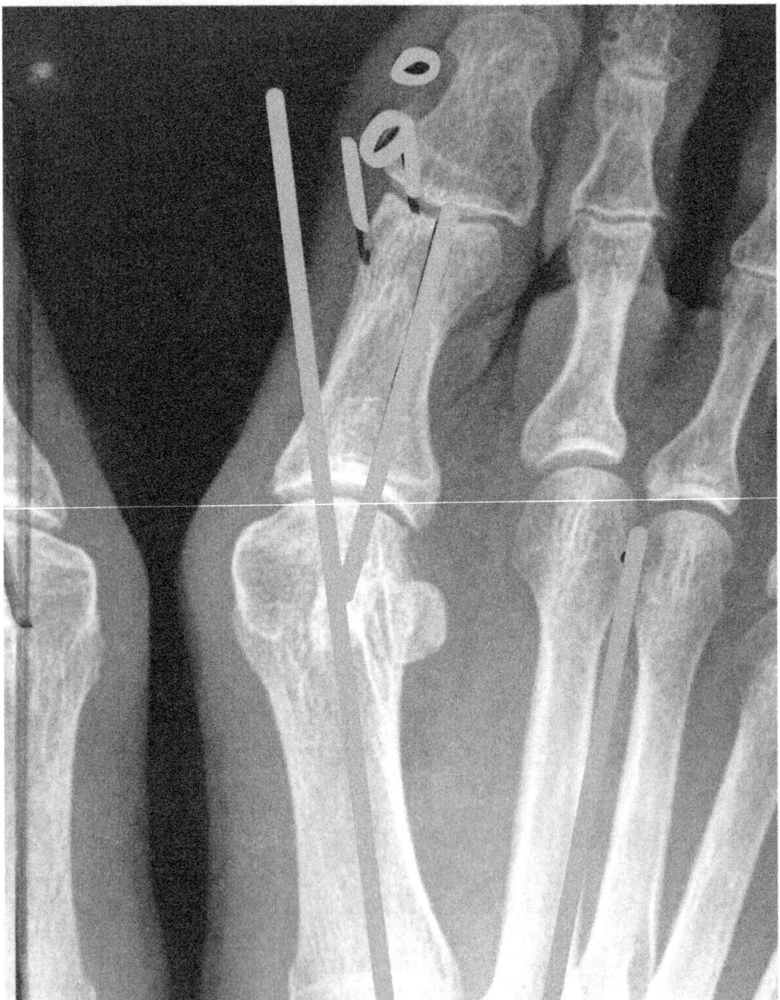

Our mission was accomplished—not only were her bunions significantly reduced, she was no longer experiencing any foot pain.

We finished the corrective phase of Pam's treatment, and then we sent her for a follow-up X-ray. On measuring the difference between the angles of deviation at Pam's big toe (bunion), we saw that the treatment had straightened the right toe by 6 degrees.

The great news is that with minimal ongoing treatment, we will be able to further straighten the bunion until there is no deviation whatsoever. In actual fact, given that the ideal reading is 15 degrees, we are confident that her toes will be straight in no time.

Well done, Pam! In Pam's case, there was no need for either expensive surgery, or for a change in her footwear!

Allison's Case

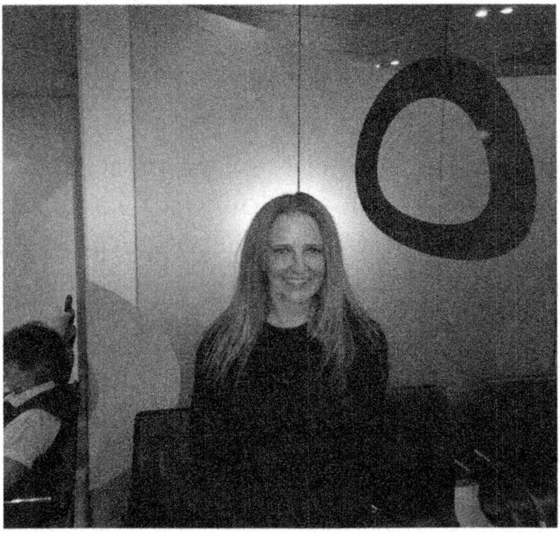

Meet Alison, a patient with a classic case of bunions and plantar fasciitis. In Alison's case, both conditions were primarily caused by the misalignment of her lower limb, which affected the way she walked and ran.

Alison had advanced bunions bilaterally (the big toe turned inwards), and was suffering from plantar fasciitis. When we met her, she was extremely frustrated because she was accustomed to being active, but was now unable to exercise. The problems with her feet were also making her job as a theatre nurse increasingly difficult.

It is always our top priority to help our patients achieve their goals. Alison's main goal was to be able to run again. She was surprised to hear that we could straighten her bunion too, as it was quite advanced.

After medically assessing Alison's case during our initial consultation, we referred her for an X-ray. This was Alison's initial X-ray. As you can see, it shows a bunion angle of 29 degrees on the left big toe and 34 degrees on the right. The ideal angle is 12–15 degrees. We definitely had some work to do on a few fronts. After discussion, we decided on a course of foot mobilisation in conjunction with strengthening exercises.

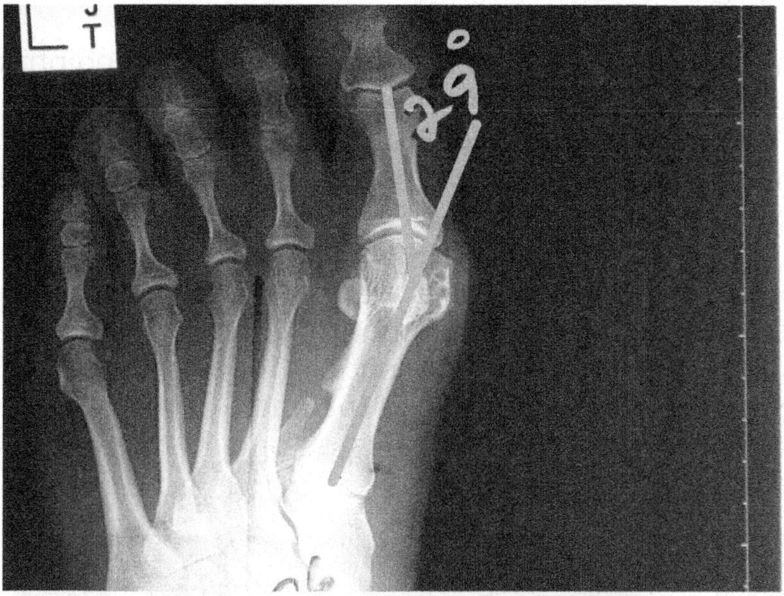
29°

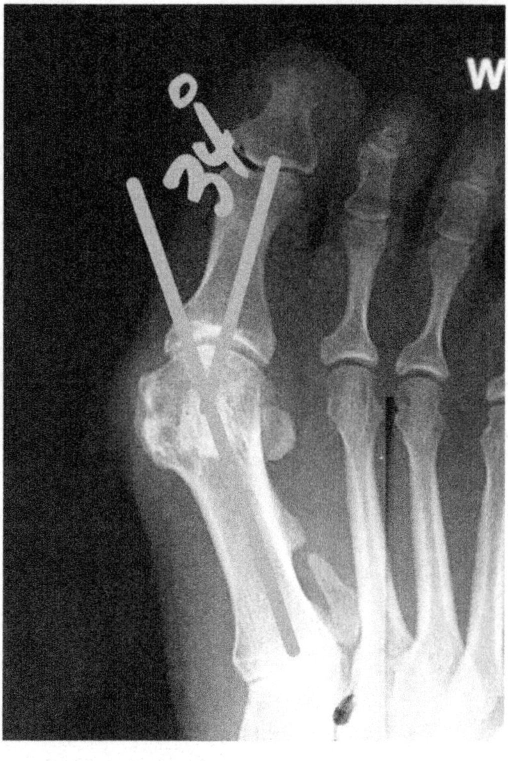
34°

Running again in under a month!

To her credit, Alison was enthusiastic about the appointments and the exercises. She reported a significant reduction in pain in both the bunion and the plantar fasciitis, to the point where we decided she could start running again. During that time, Alison commented that she could see her 'big toe straightening'.

In Alison's case, the four weeks were the most intense aspect of the treatment, with a reduction in frequency of visits after that. As with all our patients, we sent Alison for a follow-up X-ray to measure her results. We found the angle of her bunion was down to 23 degrees on the left big toe and 27 degrees on the right—a huge improvement.

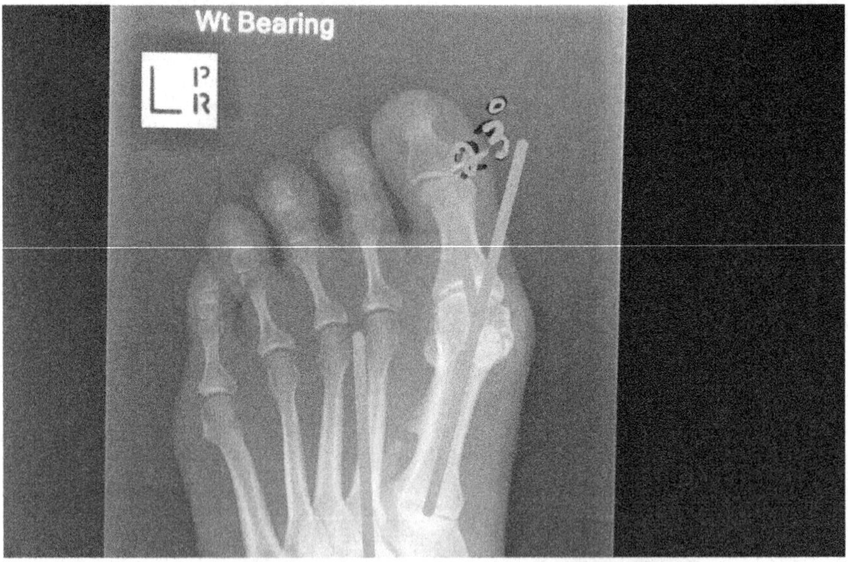

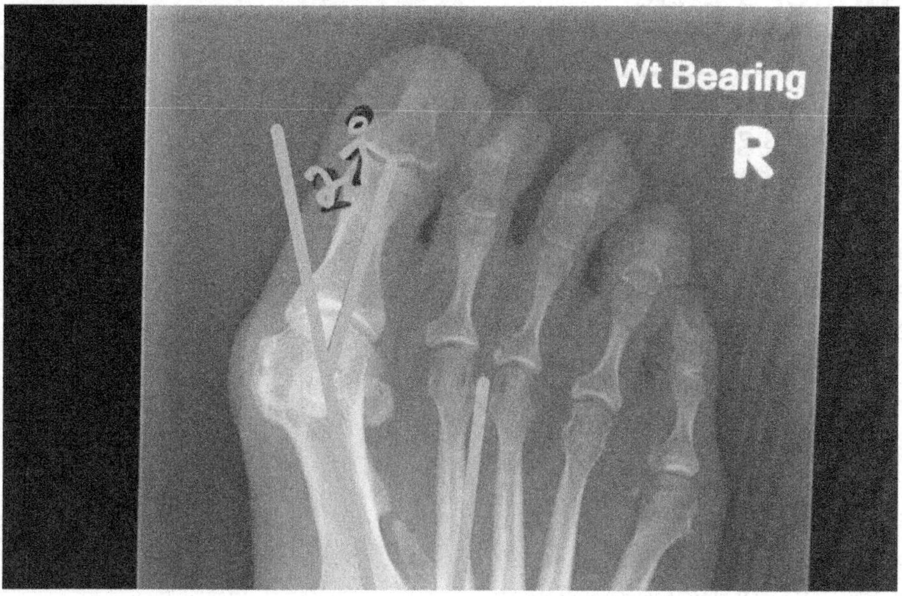

Most importantly, Alison is now pain free! I believe she is currently training for a marathon and wears the shoes she loves. This is because we addressed the alignment of Alison's foot, which was the underlying cause—no Band-aid solutions.

Jennifer's Case

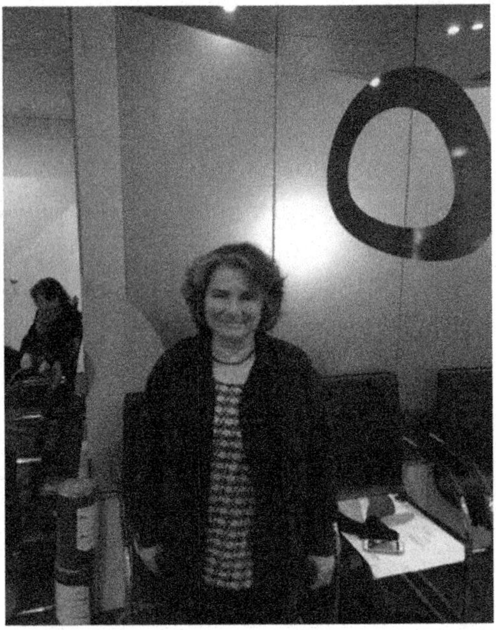

Jennifer attended Alternative Foot Solutions due to a significant bunion deviation on both sides, and due to pain in her forefoot, underneath her second metatarsal. As a result, the second toe was starting to become raised and claw on its way to a hammer toe.

Jennifer was highly motivated to get her foot fixed, and she was pleasantly surprised to hear that we were confident that not only could we treat the pain under the ball of her foot, we could also correct the bunion deviation. What was more surprising was that we could achieve both of these outcomes without her needing to change her footwear or limit her lifestyle.

After establishing Jennifer's personal goals, we medically assessed her case during our initial consultation, which included an X-ray. This was Jennifer's initial X-ray. As you can see below, her initial X-ray shows that her bunion angle was 37 degrees. The ideal angle is 12 -15 degrees.

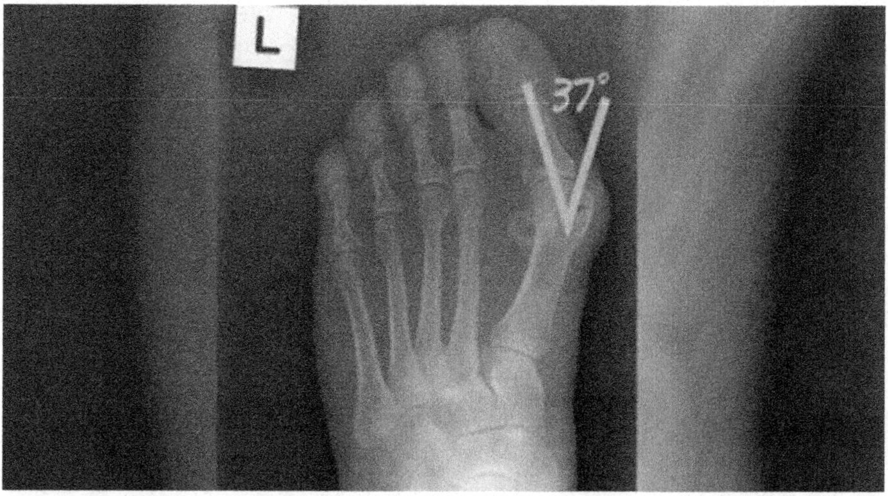

To her credit, Jennifer was enthusiastic about the appointments and the exercises. Within four weeks, there was a significant reduction in the pain in the ball of the foot.

In Jennifer's case, the four weeks were the most intense aspect of the treatment, with a reduction in frequency of visits after that.

As we do with all our bunion corrections, we sent Jennifer for a follow up X-ray to measure her results. We managed to get down to 29 degrees, which is a huge improvement.

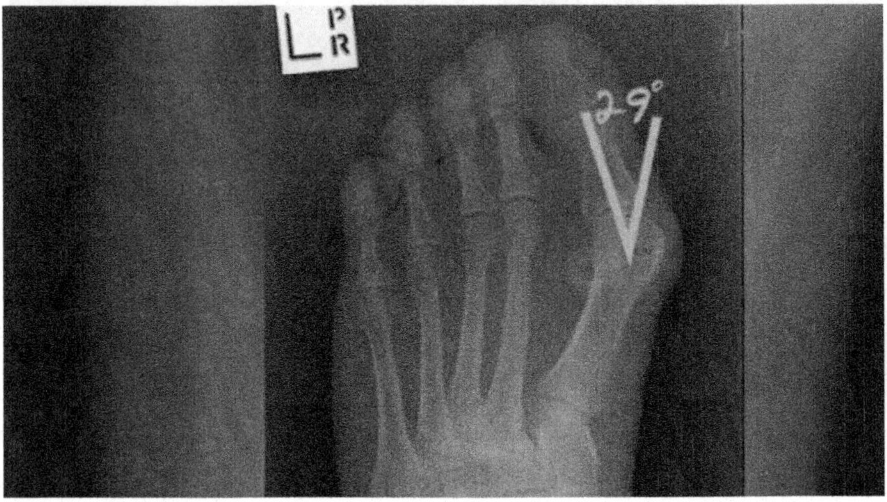

In Jennifer's case, we didn't think an improvement like this was possible up until a few years ago.

Yet, we have worked diligently on improving our technique, and the fact that approximately 70% of our patient load is bunion correction has afforded us an invaluable opportunity to hone and perfect our technique.

We have successfully treated thousands of bunions between us at Alternative Foot Solutions, and we believe that there is a better alternative to surgery or constant pain due to a bunion. We feel the sooner the bunion is treated, the better the long term result.

So, what do you have to lose, apart from your bunion?

Call now on 8966 9300, or contact us on info@alternativefootsolutions.com.au

CHAPTER FIVE

Safer Ways to Fix a Bunion

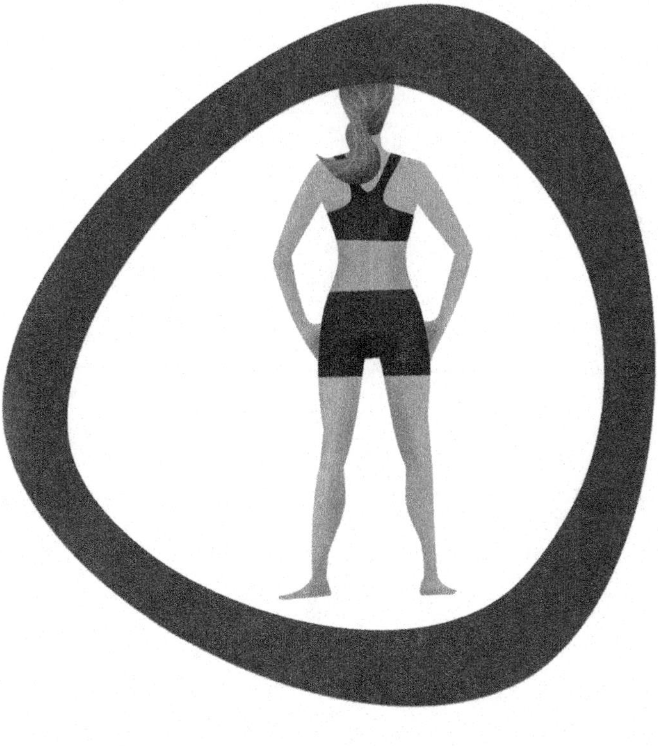

How does foot mobilisation therapy work?

1. As your podiatrist, I use foot mobilisation therapy to gently and painlessly take the joints of your feet through their natural range of motion, and then that actually corrects their position.

2. I then teach you a few quick and easy podiatry exercises to strengthen the relevant structures and muscles in your feet. The exercises generally take no more than five minutes per day, and most can be done while you do something else, like take taking a shower.

3. Unlike orthotics, which are effective only when in use, foot mobilisation therapy changes the structure of your feet—so you're healing every minute of the day.

How do I know whether foot mobilisation therapy will work for me?

1. Book an initial podiatric assessment (of about 20 minutes) with me at Alternative Foot Solutions so that we can discuss whether foot mobilisation therapy is the best option for you.

2. If we need more information, we may send you for further examinations (such as an X-ray).

3. I always recommend the treatment that will best fit with your lifestyle.

Alternative Foot Solutions – A Sydney-based Podiatry Service (Your Sydney Podiatrist)

Alternative Foot Solutions is based in a Sydney podiatry clinic that specialises in foot mobilisation therapy for the treatment of a wide range of foot pain, biomechanical, or and body movement issues. Assessment and treatment techniques combine a mixture of mainstream podiatry treatments with foot mobilisation and acupuncture, employing a holistic approach to treating foot problems pain.

Top Tips to Support the Process of Fixing Your Bunions

Follow both tips to fix your bunions!

Top tip 1—Heel Raise (Foot Extension)

This exercise helps to strengthen the muscles around the joints and will help to straighten you toes.

How to do this exercise:

1. Stand with your feet comfortably apart.

2. Come onto the balls of your feet about 3/4 as high as you can go. Hold for 3 seconds.

Perform 10 sets, twice daily.

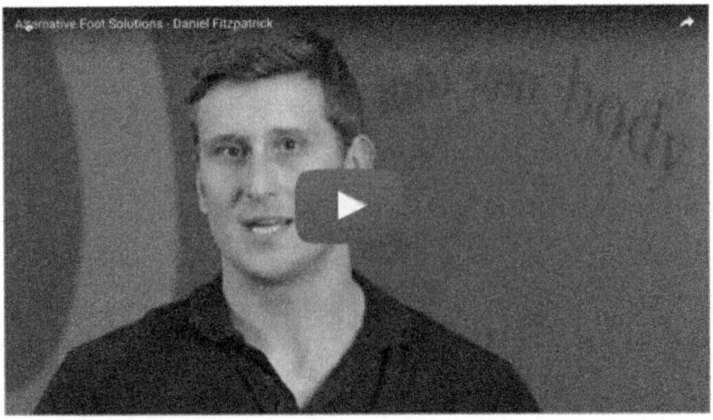

Go to www.alternativefootsolutions.com.au for videos on how to do this exercise

Top Tip 2—Get An Assessment NOW!

Exercises alone will not fix your bunions. It is important to correct the joints of your feet and address the underlying issues as well. The longer you leave it, the closer you are to the deformity and surgery—not to mention foregoing the chance to wear the shoes you love. We can fix your bunions without surgery, without pain, and without changing your shoes!

Mention this book to receive your initial assessment free (valued at $100). Get a full assessment on us.

Call now on (02) 8966 9300. or visit
www.alternativefootsolutions.com.au

Orthotics don't fix bunions but we do!

A paper was recently presented at a podiatry conference I attended. The conference topic was about measuring the validity of orthotic treatment for bunions. Not surprisingly, the research found that orthotic therapy did nothing to improve bunions.

Now don't get me wrong: I actually do think that orthotics are a great therapy for a number of issues, but it amazes me that podiatrists still use orthotics in the treatment of bunions, particularly since there is now compelling evidence that orthotics aren't corrective, but are accommodative instead.

I think it's completely dishonest for podiatrists to use orthotics in the treatment of bunions, particularly considering that people think orthotics will not only stop their bunion, but correct it. One has to ask whether this in the best interests of the patient or simply an exercise to benefit cash flow. Just last night, I did an assessment on a 14-year-old female who was prescribed orthotics to fix her bunion subsequent to being told that they would help her bunion.

Thankfully, her mum looked us up after 18 months at the stage when her bunion was getting worse and also causing pain. I admit that the orthotic will slow the development of a bunion while the patient is wearing the orthotic, but who can wear an orthotic 24 hours a day 7 days a week, especially a 14-year-old girl?

To correct a bunion, you need to correct the underlying cause. This is where Foot mobilisation Therapy (FMT) comes in. FMT changes the alignment of your joints by gently guiding them back into a corrected position, and we then combine this with exercises that are specific to bunions in order to reinforce this corrected position. This treatment regime addresses the underlying cause so that the change is long-term, and the problem is fixed forever.

Why night splints are a waste of Time!

There are hundreds of products on the market that claim to fix your bunion. The problem is I don't think I've found any that work and I would have to say we've tried a lot of them out there. The primary problem with night splints is that they don't address the underlying cause, which is the way that you stand or walk.

We spoke in previous chapters about the magnitude of force that goes through your big toe; the problem is that your big toe is being pushed out of alignment with double your weight for most of the day. Therefore, a small, comfortable device that is worn when you're not weight-bearing is unlikely to work.

There is one device that we have found does work, but it only works in conjunction with foot mobilisation therapy. However, if it's used by itself, it doesn't fix your bunion.

Foot Mobilisation Technique (FMT)

FOOT PAIN

We challenge traditional treatments with great results!
We believe that we can correct the underlying cause of your foot and leg problems without you having to resort to orthotics, compromise on your fashionable footwear choices, or impede your activity.

We challenge traditional treatments, and can achieve treatment outcomes that previously required orthotics or, in many cases, even surgery.

FOOT MOBILISATION

Foot mobilisation is a hands-on technique that gently corrects the alignment of the lower leg in order to address the underlying cause of pain or misalignment. It is corrective rather than accommodative, so improvement takes place continuously; that is, 24 hours a day, seven days a week.These changes are then supported with exercises that can be done at home in just a few minutes per day. Foot mobilisation can be used as a treatment option in most cases of foot and leg pain, or misalignment.

These conditions may include but are not restricted to:

» Bunions
» Heel pain
» Plantar fascitis
» Heel spurs
» Clawed or hammer toes
» Morton’s neuroma
» Pain when standing
» Aching feet
» Osteoarthritis
» Rheumatoid arthritis

- Poor balance
- Kid's feet (growing pains)
- Pain when wearing heels or fashionable footwear
- Knee pain

Foot Mobilisation: what is it and where did it come from?

Foot Mobilisation Therapy (FMT) is a technique that improves the function and alignment of the foot through gentle mobilisation in conjunction with exercises. Treatment is tailored to the patient, depending on the level of care needed.

Unlike other treatments, FMT does not prescribe footwear to patients. It allows freedom of choice when it comes to shoes and to activity, and it improves quality of life.
Foot mobilisation addresses the cause of the issue and helps to render the patient self-sufficient in the long term.

The practice of FMT is a specifically developed form of manual therapy aimed at improving your foot and leg functionality. FMT targets joints of your foot and ankle, which may be stiff, poorly aligned or dysfunctional, and it aims to gradually restore the way they work. This is achieved via a series of hands-on treatment sessions, in conjunction with a specific exercise regime that we prescribe for you.

Where did FMT originate?

Used extensively in the areas of physiotherapy, chiropractic and osteopathy, FMT originated from a type of treatment called manipulative therapy.

Foot mobilisation techniques have evolved from combining the podiatric biomechanical understanding of foot and leg function with the manual therapeutic experience of physiotherapy and chiropractic.

Dr John Martin Hiss from North America was the pioneer of manipulative techniques for feet and ankles. With the help of a collaborative team of MDs, osteopaths, podiatrists and chiropractors, Dr Hiss set up clinics across the US in the 1920s to treat foot pain.

A student of Dr Hiss, Dr Harvey Lampell, further refined the technique and taught the improved version to Ted Jedynak. Jedynak worked extensively with Lampell before refining the technique even further, and he went on to introduce FMT to Australia.

At Alternative Foot Solutions, our practitioners have worked and studied with Ted Jedynak to learn these techniques. Daniel and Lachlan are now involved in teaching the techniques to other practitioners.

"We use these techniques together with a variety of other mobilisation techniques that have been learned from a number of musculo-skeletal physicians. We are the only clinic in NSW to specialise in foot mobilisation therapy, and we have over 15 years of experience in this area.

As they say, "The proof is in the pudding", and our excellent results speak for themselves. Unlike other podiatry-based practices, we work exclusively in the area of FMT to treat foot and associated pain.

Our unique approach differs to that of other podiatrists in the following ways:

» Our practices were established solely to deliver FMT to you; no other clinic in New South Wales does this.
» Our practitioners apply FMT to work with the cause of your foot and leg pain. We provide long-term care solutions, which require treating the origin of your pain.

- No surgery, medication or orthotics are employed in your treatment.
- FMT promotes your body's natural repair process. Because there are no orthotics, you don't need special shoes, artificial soles or shoe inserts, which limit your choice of footwear.
- We provide post-treatment care involving useful information and easily implemented exercises that maintain the repair process and prevent future pain and problems.

- Because the treatment environment is also a key component in the effectiveness of your care, our centres have a warm, relaxed and friendly atmosphere.

Common Questions About Treatment

How can I decrease my dependence on orthotics?

Foot mobilisation podiatry coaxes your feet and body back to health by encouraging the joints of your feet to move through their natural range of motion. This corrects the position of your feet with movement and provides permanent physiological improvements.

Unlike orthotics, which only work when you wear them, foot mobilisation changes the structure of your feet so your condition continues to improve with time.

How does it work?

The treatment is a gentle series of movements through the joints of your feet, guided by the podiatrist's hands in a controlled movement. These movements may also include your hips and knees.

Does the therapy hurt?

Generally—no. Sometimes initial mobilisations may be uncomfortable due to restriction within a joint but generally, the treatment is pain free.

Do I have to change my shoes?

No; not at all. This is the big advantage of foot mobilisation therapy (FMT). Because the change is intrinsic, it does not restrict your choice of footwear. FMT is not reliant on devices like orthotics.

Should I change my activity?

Generally, no. We actually encourage you to continue normal levels of activity. This allows us to monitor the treatment's effectiveness.

Do I have to continue the treatment forever?

Our goal is to make you as self-sufficient as possible after the initial treatment period. The advantage is that we focus on the cause of your pain by improving the alignment of your joints, and strengthening the muscles supporting those joints rather than trying to accommodate the problem, as other styles of treatment do.

CHAPTER SIX

Post Treatments Tips

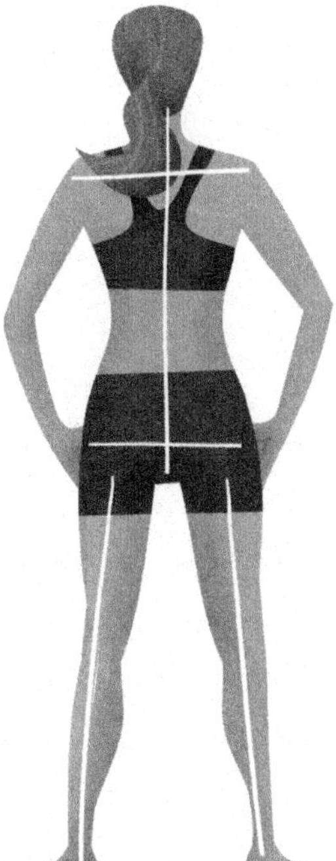

When fixing a bunion, these exercises are only really effective after or when combined with foot mobilisation therapy.

Unfortunately, exercises on their own simply won't work when treating a bunion. Furthermore, relapse prevention work can be helpful: It can be beneficial to have your joints mobilised regularly over the course of your life so that recidivism is discouraged.

All joints respond well to maintenance. It's neither today nor next year that your foot will suddenly go back to the way it was after a course of treatment of treatment, but your job is to get the best possible result forever.

How often maintenance treatment is indicated varies from person to person, and also, it varies as a function of the nature of people's movement patterns.

Heel Raises

Why do this exercise? This exercise helps to strengthen the muscles around the joints that have been adjusted by the practitioner.

The stronger these muscles are, the longer your adjustments will hold, which will, in turn, help to strengthen the foot muscles relevant to keeping your bunion straight.

How to do this exercise:

1. Stand with your feet comfortably apart.
2. Come onto the balls of your feet about 3/4 as high as you can go

How often? Hold for 3 seconds

10 sets, twice daily

Bunion Exercise (Adductor Hallucis)

Why Do This Exercise? This exercise will strengthen the muscle that moves your big toe from side to side. This will assist in slowing the progress of a bunion deformity, and it will help with the realignment of the big toe.

How To Do This Exercise?

» Sit on the edge of a chair with your feet on the ground.
» Relax your feet and legs.
» Move your big toe away from your other toes with your hand, keeping the muscles relaxed.
» Keep the toe in this position by tensing the muscles and pushing the inside and outside edge of your toe/foot into the floor.

NOTE: There may not be much movement of the big toe; perhaps, there will be movement of only a few millimetres. The muscles need to be relaxed until the big toe is in position. You can use something to put the big toe in position if you can't reach it, e.g. a ruler or a wooden spoon.

As part of our treatment process, we also use a type of toe spacer. This spacer wouldn't really achieve much in the way of straightening your bunion if it is not in used in conjunction with foot mobilisation therapy. However, we have found it improves our results both during the corrective phase of treatment, and also during the maintenance phase.

CHAPTER SEVEN

Why choose Us?

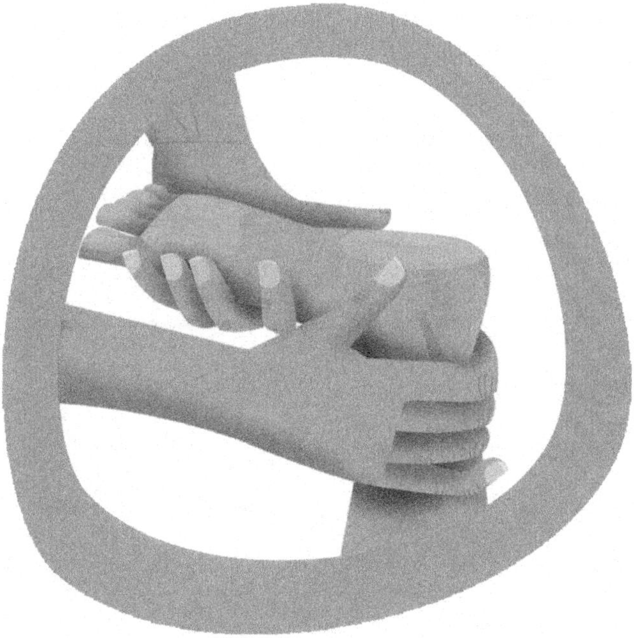

Our techniques challenge traditional treatments and challenge their limitations. Particularly when it comes to bunions!

We believe that people should be able to be pain free, and that they should be able to fix their foot problems including bunions without having to resort to drugs, surgery or even orthotics.

In fact, we have a success rate of over 90% in getting people out of orthotics. And I can't remember the last time we couldn't straighten someones bunion.

We specialise in foot mobilisation therapy, which is a gentle hands-on technique that corrects the alignment of the foot and leg, and removes the compensations that are occurring and lead to pain.

This means natural, effective healing. This treatment helps your body to help itself. Because we do things differently, we thought we'd let you know what to expect when you visit our clinic.

When you do come in for an initial assessment, you will be seen by one of our practitioners who has a very specialised skill set that has been refined and developed over a period of 13 years.

In fact our practitioners now teach this technique to other health practitioners in Australia.We are the only clinic of our nature in New South Wales.

During the initial consultation, we will undergo a detailed clinical evaluation of your condition to determine whether or not our services are the best option for you. If we feel that what we have to offer isn't the best fit for you, we'll tell you that right up front.

We may need to use X-rays for diagnostic purposes. This is a well-developed technique that allows us to pinpoint and address the underlying cause of your problem so that we can maximise treatment benefits for you.

With modern imagining techniques, the level of radiation for an X-ray is extremely low; in fact, it's about the equivalent of watching a football game on TV.

We have treated thousands of people over the years and we are extremely proud of our success rate with this treatment particuarly when it comes to straightening bunions.

So, if you're looking for a natural treatment option that doesn't limit footwear, will help you avoid surgery, and help you to avoid having to wear orthotics, then FMT should be considered.

Are you frustrated with limitations when it comes to treating bunions with traditional foot treatments, such as orthotics, surgery, pain killers and a lack of fashionable footwear options? If you're asking these questions, I can relate, because 14 years ago, this is exactly why I decided to specialise in FMT.

In fact, it was my frustration with traditional methods that led me to start Alternative Foot Solutions, which was and still is the only clinic in New South Wales to specialise in foot mobilisation .

Our vision is to offer our clients a better alternative when it comes to care of their lower limbs.

We will alleviate your foot pain, get you moving and give you the freedom to wear the shoes you love. At Alternative Foot Solutions, we believe in helping people to improve the quality of their lives.

We want to alleviate your fix your bunion, keep you active, and give you freedom of choice when it comes to what shoes you want to wear. We want to keep you out of orthotics.

We're particularly accomplished at helping fashion conscious women with their leg and feet problems, but don't want to compromise their lifestyle choices.

We fix your foot issues, without compromising on footwear, activity, and without having to resort to surgery.

You see, we do things a little differently. For one, we employ advanced assessment techniques that are measurable and give objective feedback to you, the client.

We show all our patients the correction that has occurred over the course of their treatment via X-ray, and we measure the improvements via objective measurements.

Our techniques challenge traditional treatments and their limitations so that our client gets the best possible outcome. In fact, we have a 93% success rate at getting people out of their orthotics.

We approach our level of care this way because we believe that traditional treatments limit the results that we've found are possible by using our foot mobilisation techniques.

We believe that traditional therapies, such as orthotics, do not address the underlying cause of the problem. We get to the cause and our methods offer a far superior solution that will optimise your lifestyle and your fashion choices.

A crucial point is that we are on a mission to treat the underlying cause, not just the symptom.

Not only will you receive improvements in aches and pains, you will have the best opportunity to receive long term health and well-being.

Unlike other health services that offer band-aid solutions, which are short term at best, we are wanting to achieve the best long term outcome for you and your body. Remember that everything works best when it's in the right position.

This is particularly relevant for your feet and legs, because when these joints are in the wrong position or have a significant level of misalignment, the soft tissues are forced to compensate.

The discomfort you're feeling is as a result of compensation. So, what we want to address is the underlying cause, which is that your joints aren't in the right position.

Think about it: If your joints are misaligned it leads the articular surfaces of your bones to wear unevenly. This leads to painful inflammation in the soft tissues, and even irreversible damage in the form of osteoarthritis.

Unfortunately if your have a bunion forming and don't correct the misalignment then it s only a matter of time.

We don't argue with women about the type of footwear they should wear. We don't need to anymore, because we now have a solution to give them what they want for their problem feet.

Traditional podiatry is effective, but Foot Mobilisation Therapy (FMT) is even more effective, without an orthotic in sight. That's because orthotics work like reading glasses—they're only effective when in use. FMT changes the structure of your body, so you're healing every minute of the day.

And orthotics don't fit inside your Jimmy Choos.

We've learnt that with orthotics, the issue is always that women have extreme difficulty wearing and using them due to footwear limitations and especially not when treating bunions.

As qualified medical professionals, we know feet, but we also understand a woman's desire to wear beautiful shoes. We help women achieve their desire without harming their feet.

Alternative Foot Solutions specialises in alternative but effective ways to treat your feet, without invasive surgery or orthotics. The benefits to you are the elimination of pain, permanent physiological improvements to your body, and the ability to wear the footwear of your choice.

Mention this book to receive your initial assessment free (valued at $100). Get a full assessment on us.

Call now on (02) 8966 9300. or visit www. alternativefootsolutions.com.au

CPSIA information can be obtained
at www.ICGtesting.com
Printed in the USA
BVOW06s1958160517
484307BV00009B/280/P

9 781945 173851